The Child's World

New approaches to the hor
treatment of children

Saltire Books   *Saltire Books Limited, Glasgow, Scotland*

The Child's World

New approaches to the
homeopathic treatment of children

by

Linda Johnston MD

Saltire Books *Saltire Books Limited, Glasgow, Scotland*

Published by Saltire Books Ltd

18–20 Main Street, Busby, Glasgow G76 8DU, Scotland
books@saltirebooks.com   www.saltirebooks.com

 is a registered trademark

Saltire Books

First published 2010

Typeset by Type Study, Scarborough, UK in 10 on 12$^1/_2$ Dyadis
Printed by Information Press Ltd, Eynsham, Oxford, UK

ISBN-13: 978 1 95 590651 0

For Saltire
Project Development: Lee Kayne
Editorial: Steven Kayne
Design: Phil Barker

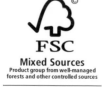

FSC

Mixed Sources
Product group from well-managed
forests and other controlled sources

Cert no. SA-COC-002048
www.fsc.org
© 1996 Forest Stewardship Council

Forest Stewardship Council is a non-profit international organisation established to promote the responsible management of the world's forests. Products carrying the FSC label are independently certified to assure consumers that they are sourced from forests managed to meet the social, economic and ecological needs of present and future generations.

CONTENTS

Acknowledgements   ix
About the Author   xi

1   Introduction   1
2   Traditional Approaches to Children's Cases   7
3   New Approaches to Children's Cases   19
4   Childhood Development   33
5   Methods and Techniques   77
6   The Source Revealed   109
7   Mother and Child   137
8   The Child's Environment   175
9   Parents   191

    Index   203

Dedication

This book is dedicated to my father

Gerald F. Johnston

ACKNOWLEDGEMENTS

No one deserves more credit for making this book happen than Sverre Klemp, former idea man at Thieme Verlagsgruppe publishers, the great folks who bring the homeopathy world LINKS every quarter. Writing another book on the homeopathic treatment of children would not have been so intriguing to me had not Sverre's vision included the innovative idea of focusing on the new and successful trends in homeopathy that have arisen in the last decade. After single-handedly getting the ball rolling, we began to work together. In the early months of our discussions about his brainchild, his contributions, convictions and exemplary insights into both what was absent from the literary marketplace as well as what would best serve homeopaths increased my respect and admiration for his seemingly bottomless talent and perspicacity. As a result of our collaboration, we developed his initial inspiration into what you are reading now. It has been a process of immense enjoyment and creativity and for that, I have Sverre to thank.

As the book took its final form, Steven and Lee Kayne of Saltire Books played a greater part. It has been their experience, creativity and commitment to producing not only worthwhile and useful books on homeopathy, but beautifully formatted and designed books that has garnished my deep gratitude and appreciation. The difference between my manuscript and the book you are holding now, with its easy-on-the-eye font, pertinent and illustrative pictures, securing binding and styling is colossal. Add to that their tireless efforts at copy editing, distribution, publicity and the many other behind the scenes activities of a publisher that generally go unnoticed, and it will be apparent why I extend my most heart-felt thanks to everyone at Saltire Books who have participated in the creation of this book. I want to make a special mention and give fond appreciation to the darlings of the pictures, Alex, Eilidh and Zak, and their parents for allowing us to use their images. Each pictures does more than add a thousand words, as the adage goes, to exemplify the content of this book.

Dr. Sunil Anand also deserves extra special mention. I owe him an enormous debt of gratitude. His participation in this book actually started many years ago when I first began to learn about the treatment of children under his amazing tutelage. Sunil has a well-deserved worldwide reputation as the leading expert in children cases and it has always been a source of great satisfaction that I have had the privilege of learning from him over the years. His combination of a calm and gentle manner, amazing perception and vast knowledge is a benchmark for any of us who treat children to aspire. Dr. Anand's contribution of cases with comments and analysis have made this book far better and instructive than it otherwise would have been. As you read and learn from his cases in this book, I am sure you will gain as much as I have.

Another contributor, Rachel Lipman Mostow, has a special place in my heart. You will read about her experiences in her own words in chapter nine. I have treated her and her four children for many years. It is people like Rachel that make being a homeopath even more amazing and wonderful than it already is. Her intelligence, perception and dedication to her values and her family are worthy of everyone's admiration. From the first visit, she demonstrated an eagerness infused with discerning intelligence to learn about what was happening to herself and her children, what homeopathy could do and how it did it. Over the years, she has developed keen insight and an ability to observe and understand her children that is a delight to behold. I thank her not only for her contribution to the book, but for the many enjoyable years of working together.

There are many others who have made this book possible and my deepest and most sincere appreciation goes out to each and every one. I am most grateful to Divya Chhabra, Rajan Sankaran, Jayesh Shah, Sujit Chatterjee, Sudhir Balbota and all my other teachers for contributing so much to my understanding and abilities as a homeopath.

Last but not least, I want to thank my wonderful husband, Frans Vermeulen. His support and loving kindness has made every day, not just book-writing days, bountiful beyond measure.

Linda Johnston MD
February 2010

ABOUT THE AUTHOR

Dr Linda Johnston has been a active member of the homeopathic community worldwide since the inception of her homeopathic practice in 1986. After completing her medical training from the University of Washington, USA in 1979, she had one further year in family medicine. She started her own private medical practice in 1981. Linda began her homeopathic training in 1986, and began practicing the same year. Her main focus has always been on the clinical practice of homeopathy, which she continues to this day.

Contributing to the homeopathic community through writing and teaching are both important to Linda. From 1991–1996, she developed and taught a two-year homeopathy curriculum in 4 different US cities to train licensed medical practitioners. She is also a well-known teacher internationally.

Author of numerous articles for homeopathy journals, Linda is also the author of *Additions to the Homeopathic Repertory from Kent's lectures on Homeopathic Materia Medica* (Christine Kent Agency, 1990) as well as a popular book for the general public, *Everyday Miracles: Homeopathy in Action* (Christine Kent Agency, 1991). Since her debut public lecture in 1987, she has made hundreds of radio, television appearances, in addition to print media interviews educating the public about homeopathy.

Linda's current projects include co-authoring, with her husband Frans Vermeulen, a comprehensive work on plants and plant families, the first two volumes of which are due for publication in 2010.

1

INTRODUCTION

The approach to treating children

In every homeopathy seminar that I have ever attended, and there have been many, inevitably the question is asked, 'What about treating children?' This question is made possible by the notion that treating children is fundamentally different than treating adults. People are people all over the world, and homeopathy treats everyone, all ages, all cultures and all stages of life in basically the same way. Yet, undeniably there are differences in childhood and these do have an impact on the approach to treating children.

One obvious distinction that confronts homeopaths is that children have either no verbal ability, or a limited ability to express themselves or communicate about their physical or emotional concerns. Considering that the homeopathic methodology depends on understanding the individual patient's experience to be able to prescribe correctly, homeopaths wonder how it is possible to obtain the necessary information from a non-verbal patient. This is just one of many distinctive characteristics about childhood which requires special skills and insights. Relying on observation alone as a means of gathering information is not useful unless one knows what to look for and how to understand what one sees.

This book assists the homeopath to develop a deeper understanding of the nature of childhood, the developmental stages and how the world looks from the child's perspective.

Most homeopaths treat children as some portion of their practice. Some homeopaths' practices are mostly children. Whether one child a year is treated or the greater part of their time is spent with children patients, all homeopaths want to prescribe successfully for each and every one of them. Anyone in practice for any length of time will naturally develop their own style, preferred methods, ideas and approach to patients. As homeopaths continue to learn and gain more experience, their personal style evolves. This occurs while still maintaining a firm stand on the foundation of basic principles in common to all homeopaths.

From the beginning student of homeopathy to the seasoned practitioner, all can benefit from more knowledge and skills. The ideas in this book are designed to broaden the foundation by expanding the fundamental principles that underpin your work as well as enhancing your skills with new perspectives and techniques. In other words, from wherever you are now, this book should help you journey further into the realm of successful understanding of, and prescribing for, children. Starting with the traditional methods, the book moves forward to explore and encompass the new ideas and methods in homeopathy and how they are successfully applied to children's cases.

What is the treatment goal?

Everyone makes a decision about how they want to care for their health, and parents choose for their children. Some people choose to subscribe to the conventional medical ideas and methods while others choose no medical care at all. Others decide to adopt homeopathy for their medical care. These choices not only affect what happens when a person becomes ill, but also how they live their life and take care of themselves. In a word, choosing homeopathy for one's healthcare is a part of a lifestyle based on a view of life, which appreciates the interconnectedness of all life, all nature and every aspect of each person. Homeopathy is part of life, not a detour from it.

The first step in any therapeutic situation, even before considering a particular method, is to have a firm understanding of the goal of treatment. As homeopaths, what is it we are trying to do? What is our mission statement? For the current topic, what is the goal in treating a child with homeopathy? Are we solely interested in getting rid of symptoms? Do we want to simply eliminate the fever, resolve the inflamed ear, stop an asthma attack or soothe the fussy child? Do we have a larger, more comprehensive goal?

This relevant issue is grounded in ideas about health, disease and homeopathy. Understanding about health and disease comes first before a realistic goal can be formulated. This understanding is fundamental to any method of therapeutics. What is disease? What is health? What is a healthy child? For homeopaths, thinking about these questions is not a new endeavour. From the beginning, the study of homeopathy challenged us with these philosophical and methodological inquiries. Turning our thoughts to these issues has never been mere idle speculation or a pointless exercise. It is a significant and essential part of homeopathy and touches the deeper meaning and significance of health and disease for a deeper level of healing.

Hahnemann states that a homeopath must clearly and accurately determine what is sick in the patient. This profoundly insightful mandate can be fulfilled only when we know exactly how health should appear. Then it is possible to perceive the contrast between the existing ill state and the healthy state that we wish to achieve for the patient. This is equally true when treating children. Therefore, the first step towards enhancing the child's health is to understand fully all the normal changes taking place throughout childhood, the stages of a child's innate healthy developmental process and how the healthy child experiences life. Knowing what health is, it is possible to perceive what is sick in the child.

This may seem unnecessarily complex. After all, isn't it obvious that a child is sick when he has a fever, a rash, an ear infection, a cough or colic? Our goal, however, is not simply to eliminate these individual symptoms, but to restore the entire child to health. To do that, the child in his totality is taken into consideration by knowing what is normal and expected at each stage of a child's life.

Traditional and new methods

With the goal identified, the next step is to ask what methods are best suited to accomplish it. Generations of homeopaths have successfully treated children with traditional approaches that rely heavily on observation, behaviour patterns coupled with remedies' keynote and pathognomonic symptoms. The homeopath observes a child's behaviour directly or hears about the child from the parents, then looks for keynote symptoms or recognises the well-known patterns of common children's types. Keynote prescribing and the concept of children's types are both discussed in more detail in chapter two.

These time-honoured methods have yielded countless successful cures over many decades. In fact, it is often this success in children's problems that has led to the spread and increasing popularity of homeopathy.

With so long a tradition of successfully treating children, why is a change needed?

Despite the good results, there have always been cases that did not lend themselves to these methods, where the 'obvious' remedy, supported by keynotes, physical symptoms and matching the known child type simply did not work. The goal was not achieved.

These are the situations that have motivated homeopaths to seek to expand their existing repertoire of methods and ideas. Springing from a solid foundation, many refinements and other techniques have added to the possibilities of understanding and correctly prescribing for children. One particularly fruitful area of innovation has been the specific group of new ideas called 'source-based' or 'sensation-based' prescribing. These topics are the focus of the rest of this book, and will be referred to collectively as 'the new methods'.

Parents

Children have parents. That much is self-evident. In that light, this distinctive aspect of childhood must be considered and integrated into the treatment approach. Parental impact and influence are such an enormous part of a child's world that who the child's parents are, their values, life style and health are factors of primary importance. Even as adults, these influences remain with us. As Wordsworth aptly noted, 'The child is father of the man.'

Also self-evident is the fact that each adult was once a child, and had to experience all the childhood phases of developing, learning, growing and exploring life. For some, those childhood experiences are still very much alive and expressive. Famed American children's author and cartoonist Dr. Seuss goes so far as to say, 'Adults are obsolete children.'

All homeopaths have had adult patients whose illness involved some unincorporated childhood stage of development or traumatic event that was still overmastering their life. In treating those cases, knowledge of childhood development, stages of growth and normal milestones will be of inestimable value. Though this is a book about the treatment of children, much of what will be discussed will apply to the understanding of those adult patients whose childhoods still loom large. After all, it is never too late to have a happy childhood.

The child is the centre of an ecosystem, which usually includes parents, other caretakers, grandparents, siblings and other relatives, all of whom have an important place in the child's life and health. Sometimes there are even more than two parents, and all too often, less than two. Homeopaths who treat children are aware of the importance of the home environment and the parental influence on the health of children. Parents are people in their own right, which needs to be considered, in addition to understanding how they structure the child's universe, interact, observe and support the child. The Swiss psychiatrist Carl Gustav Jung (1875-1961) observed that the child lives in the unconscious of the parent.[1] Another way to express that is to say that the fully conscious parent encompasses the psychological state of the child. This is a way of understanding how extremely sensitive children are to parental emotions, thoughts and actions. Using the new ideas in homeopathy, this premise takes on greater significance and is discussed at length later in the book.

To understand the child as a whole person, a complete perspective on his emotional and developmental ecosystem is needed. Making an ally of the child's parents helps enormously. Parents are useful sources of information. Yet it is necessary to remember that parents' perceptions are based on their own perspective and depth of understanding. In other words, everything heard from the parents is filtered through their own values, expectations, education, preconceived ideas and, indeed, their own level of health. Sometimes the homeopath hears more about a parent's case than the child's! Even if a parent is not a patient already, this is still useful information to help become more aware of the environment in which the child lives. The caution is that it is necessary to be able to differentiate the parent's own state from their information relating to the child, and understand how to coordinate all that information in its useful place.

As is true of homeopaths, the parents also need to understand what they are seeing in their child in order to know what value it has as information about their child's well-being and what other enquiries might be helpful. Parents can assist the homeopath to help their child by knowing how to perceive him or her from a homeopathic perspective. Deputising the parents requires only that the homeopath spends time:

- offering education in basic homeopathic philosophy,
- giving an understanding of childhood development,
- encouraging them to see the whole child,
- giving an awareness of aetiologies and stresses,
- explaining what symptoms are and how to observe them.

Working together with a 'homeopathy parent' not only can significantly enhance successful treatment of the child, but it helps parents understand their child much better. Working together with parents this way is one of the great pleasures of treating children. So important is the team work with parents, that this topic will be discussed in several later chapters.

Getting started

In this introduction many of the areas that are particular and special about treating children have been mentioned. Each of these and many others are elaborated in the following chapters, all to the purpose of giving a strong foundation in the necessary information to treat children, understanding the new methods and involving parents. The homeopaths' goal is to facilitate maximum health for the children they treat. The goal of this book is to help homeopaths attain that aspiration.

Reference

1   Jung CG Psychology of the Unconscious: London: Kegan Paul Trench Trubner 1916.

2

TRADITIONAL APPROACHES TO CHILDREN'S CASES

Generations of homeopaths have successfully treated children. During the 1800s, much of the homeopathy in America was found in the Midwest region, administered by the wives and mothers in farm community families. The great expanse of America, especially in the Great Plains, meant that millions of people were without formal medical care. A trained doctor was usually one to three days' horse ride away. Homeopathy in the form of home treatment, self-help kits and books filled the breach. As was their habit, these self-sufficient farming folks took matters into their own hands. Injuries, children's diseases, fevers and other medical problems of everyday life were successfully treated with homeopathy.

During these years, a great amount of knowledge and experience with methodology was accumulated, especially in the treatment of children and childhood ailments. The basic methods, born of long experience, have formed the foundation of our current methods of treating children. Before embarking on our exploration of the newer methods in homeopathy and their application to treating children, a briefly look at these traditional methods would be appropriate. Some of those skills will also be applicable when turning to the new methods.

Children's types

One of the most familiar and popular methods of prescribing for children is identifying them by a remedy 'type'. Though not necessarily initiated by Douglas M. Borland (1885–1960), it was his booklet *Children's Types* that greatly facilitated this approach.[1] The method classifies children in one of several well-defined types, distinguished by a group of frequently identified symptoms and characteristics.

Although this method has been and is still used for adults, it is not nearly as effective for adults as it has proven to be for children. Why does prescribing for children seem to lend itself to a limited number of type categories whereas adult prescribing requires the vast array of thousands of remedies from which to choose?

There are events in peoples' lives that are shared by most other people. For example, completing one's education, finding a life partner, having children and establishing a home. Though people have similar milestones, there is an enormous variety in the ways they experience them. The kind of education, where they go to school, the number of years they attend school and their style of learning show remarkable variation. Marriage is a universal expression of human life, yet here also there exist tremendous cultural, societal and individual distinctions. There are an enormous number of different kinds of marriage celebrations from the formalised three-day Indian traditional wedding to the 1960s flower children frolicking through the woods with carefree abandon. Adults individualise everything they do and the things they do individualise them.

The same is true for their younger selves. As children, people share the universal stages of early life with other children. For example, children develop teeth, learn to walk, cope with siblings and enter school. There is a difference, however, between these childhood events and later adult events. Children bring less individualisation and more commonality to these stages of life than adults do with their milestones. This concept will now be examined further.

Individuality and commonality

At the very beginning, everyone starts as a single fertilised cell. This single cell divides into two, then four then eight and continues to divide as growth progresses. In these very early stages, this group of cells, called the blastosphere, resembles all others. Of course, the genetic material inside each cell is very individual, but those features have not yet expressed themselves. All that can be perceived is the grouping of cells that look like all other blastosphere grouping of cells. The similarities are vastly more prominent than the individual features. As embryogenesis proceeds, more and more human features emerge and finally features distinctive of an individual person are apparent. Although there is still a great deal that one newborn has in common with all other newborns, the proportion of commonalities is slightly less and more individual characteristics are expressed.

This process does not stop at birth. As the newborn grows and travels through the developmental stages, many common events are encountered and passed. The physical and emotional reactions to these tend to follow similar patterns in most children. Naturally, from the moment of birth, and actually even before, individual differences among children are readily evident. The real issue, however, is the proportion of universal characteristics and reactions as compared to the individual ones. During the early years, children experience much that is experienced by other children and in basically the same way. Child art up to age seven is remarkably similar all over the world. After that age, individual differences emerge, demonstrating cultural influences and the child artists' preferences.

When there is a high degree of common characteristics and individuality is not as dominant, then it is possible to prescribe successfully by taking the universal characteristics into account rather than focusing on the precise individuality that is necessary in adults. As the individuality emerges, so does the need to prescribe more individualistically. After age seven to eight, the child has grown into his individual self to such a degree, that type prescribing will no longer be as successful as it was. In chapter one, the changes that contribute to the development of the child's emerging self-awareness and identity were outlined. This is one area where that impacts our prescribing.

Even adults have aspects that are not individual but remain anchored in the universal. For example anyone who falls and bruises himself, takes Arnica. There is far less need for precise individualisation of prescribing because everyone bruises in a very similar fashion when they fall. After an unexpected near death fright, most everyone responds to Aconitum. The array of acute injury remedies is the same for everyone because they react to these events in a way almost exactly similar to each other. They react as part of a universal, generic experience and not out of their own specific individuality.

In addition to several basic children's types, there are other methods traditionally employed when treating children such as repertorisation and keynote prescribing (see below). Unlike the categorising into types, these methods have been successfully used in adults. Since these methods are very familiar to most homeopaths and form the mainstay of prescribing for many others, it is not necessary to give more than a brief discussion of the principles.

Repertorisation

Repertorisation is not one single method of analysing selected symptoms in comparison and combination with each other. Despite the name, repertorisation itself does not determine the outcome; the selection of symptoms to use for the analysis is the key. Therein lies the variety of approaches under the category of repertorisation. Whereas an in-depth discussion of symptom selection for traditional repertorisation is beyond the scope of this book, suffice it to say there are several ways in which this selection process is achieved. Some homeopaths focus on strange, rare or peculiar symptoms, others on the general modalities and again others on the mind characteristics. All the symptoms gleaned are combined to find the intersecting remedy common to all. Short of that ideal, the remedy most representing the array of rubrics is chosen.

From homeopathy's inception until the mid 1980s, homeopaths repertorised symptoms using paper and pencil. Rubrics were chosen and their remedy listings placed in a paper grid after which it was possible to add up the number and value of the remedies categorised there. For any of us who have done that laborious process, it quickly became apparent that our work would be made easier by careful rubric selection. The method as well as the patient determined the rubrics used. Actually, that was a very fortunate thing. The limitations of manual repertorisation helped us be very precise and careful with our rubric selection, which was all to the good. It was usual at that time to avoid all very large rubrics, limit the total number to only those that exactly fit the case and ponder the value of each one before allowing it to be included. The result was usually a handful of small to moderately sized rubrics thoughtfully chosen. The amount of careful consideration that attended the grid making had as much or more to do with the success of this method than the grid itself.

The advent of computerised repertorisation changed all that. It was possible to include rubrics that would have been far too unwieldy to use before and the number of rubrics was virtually unlimited. Somewhere along the line, the focus of the method shifted away from the careful consideration of rubrics to the grid itself. All that seemed necessary was to collect as many rubrics as possible and then let the computer do the rest. The homeopath seemed to fade in significance, as the computer took on a life of its own. Slowly, the excitement of being able to include all manner of rubrics without pre-screening has given way to the realisation of how important exacting symptom and rubric selection is to any repertorisation. Homeopathic thinking has returned to the understanding that the key feature of any repertorisation is choosing the symptoms and rubrics according to the well-defined principles of homeopathy with the computer taking its place as a powerful adjunct to the homeopaths' thinking.

Keynote prescribing

Keynote prescribing is a version of the method of seeking for the strange, rare and peculiar and elevating that symptom to the highest consideration. The quality of a useful keynote is that it is distinct, precise and highly characteristic for one single remedy. The allopathic world uses the term 'pathognomonic' to denote a sign or symptom specifically characteristic or indicative of a particular disease or condition. This concept is like seeing the Eiffel tower and knowing you are in Paris, or being certain that you are near the River Thames in London when you see Big Ben. No other locations are possible. Interestingly the Greek roots of the term mean 'skilled in diagnosis'. That certainly should give this method a boost! With such a definitive and distinctive symptom signpost, diagnoses are more skillfully made. What enables keynote prescribing is the use of rare, and singularly distinct symptoms, rather than more common, general ones.

Prescribing for children has always lent itself to keynote prescribing. Distinctive symptoms are expressed more easily and commonly in children. They generally are less able to express a variety of possibilities. They have not yet developed the vocabulary or mental aptitude and complexity to alter or co-opt the pure expressions of their state. It is as if adults have a palette of 1000 crayons to express their inner self, whereas children have the box of six primary colours. This will be discussed in later chapters because it has an impact on why the newer methods work so well in children.

Observation

Regardless of what technique is used for symptom investigation or analysis, the mainstay of prescribing is gathering useful symptoms, in other words, the case taking. For an analysis to be useful and successful, the homeopath must accurately perceive the symptoms, properly assess the validity of each symptom and prioritise their importance. This all boils down to skillful and perceptive case taking. The only way to accomplish successful case taking is to perceive and to observe. Observing is more than just looking. It is a process of watching and listening carefully and attentively, thereby gathering information with your eyes, ears, nose and mind and then detecting and registering what is significant. In other words, observing is sensory input plus thinking. Skillful observing is the bedrock of all that a homeopath does to assess the right remedy for his patients.

Short of actually closing our eyes, people are looking at the world all the time. There is an almost passive quality to looking. Thinking, on the other hand, is not necessarily so automatic or as transparent. It is often nearly impossible to tell if someone's mind is in gear or not! A person has to put forth effort to engage his mind, and when he does, it is called concentration. The following quotations show that this has long been noted:

> 'To most people nothing is more troublesome than the effort of thinking.' (British politician and diplomat James Bryce (first Viscount Bryce) 1838–1922)[2]

> 'There is no expedient that a man will not resort to in order to avoid the real effort of thinking.' (British artist Sir Joshua Reynolds, 1723–1792)[3]

Listening with the mind engaged has been termed 'active listening'. This concept can be extended with reference to case taking and called 'active observing' or 'active perceiving'. Homeopaths see and hear but also think. Their eyes 'see' but it is their mind that 'perceives'. Homeopaths do not have the luxury of allowing their mind to be in an idle mode. They must be actively alert every single minute.

There is an enormity of sensory data coming in at break-neck speed every second. A person's mind has automatic filters that eliminate the vast majority of this incoming data. It is easy to allow those filters, with their pre-set conditions, to do the processing. That is what happens most of a person's life anyway: he or she is simply not paying attention. The hard work of thinking does not let that happen; it is overriding the default mental sorting mode. No longer are the automatic neuron connections humming along passively as always. Paying attention means staying completely attentive to data that might otherwise be filtered out. Observing, thinking and concentration is a process of perceiving that of which the person would normally not be aware. So ingrained and even essential are the brain's data filtering mechanisms that it is hard work to supercede them by including what the brain normally renders undetectable.

As every homeopath working with children experiences, there are often phone calls from patients with a suddenly ill child; the cough that started after school, the fever in the middle of the night, the asthma attack, the listlessness after the afternoon nap or any one of a variety of acute onset symptoms. Taking care of children in an emergency situation, usually over the telephone or even by email, is a common occurrence. These types of child maladies can frequently be addressed over the phone by careful questioning of an observant parent. A keynote is discovered and the problem can be easily and successfully treated. Success is even more likely if the child is well known, especially when susceptibilities and family situation are already familiar to the homeopath.

The problem, however, is that by not being able to see the patient, the homeopath lacks some important and fruitful sources of information. If a picture is worth a thousand words, then certainly the visual impression of a sick child can be worth avoiding a lot of phone time and even some wrong prescriptions. Although there are occasions when the timing and circumstances of the problem make it necessary to prescribe over the phone, it is usually far better to see the patient. This brings to mind a case I had many years ago that impressed on me the importance of visual observation. No matter how skilled we are at interviewing, no matter how much materia medica we have at hand and no matter how observant and cooperative a parent is, sometimes seeing the child is the only way to prescribe correctly.

Case 2.1   Telephone consultation

Patient
I recall the case of a seven-year-old boy with a cough of three days duration. It was a nondescript cough, as so many are. It was dry, raspy with no distinct modalities.

Consultation
Even after a long time questioning both mother and child on the phone, there were no other significant symptoms, no behaviour changes and no exciting cause. There was just an annoying, intense and persistent cough. With nothing to prescribe on, it would be tempting to tell the mother to wait and let the cough resolve on its own. The intensity of the cough and its disturbing influence precluded that strategy. Despite the inconvenience, I insisted that the mother bring the child in for a visit. I am glad that I did! Just one glimpse of the child and I knew the correct remedy. It would have been impossible to determine it without seeing the child for myself. That split second glance made all the difference between success and failure. I saw tiny petechiae on the child's eyelids.

Choice of remedy
Coughing with ecchymosis leads to only one conclusion: Arnica. Support for this is found in the rubrics

- EYE: Ecchymosis: from coughing
- EYE: Ecchymosis: Lids

Arnica is one of only two remedies in either rubric listed in Kent's Repertory[4]. On the phone, I doubt I would have thought to ask if there were any tiny red dots on the child's eyelids and it is highly doubtful the mother, observant though she was, would have thought to mention them. Yet, this unusual, rare and distinctive feature of the child, not of the cough, was the key to a successful result. Indeed, one single dose of Arnica 200c cleared up the cough immediately.

All homeopaths encounter circumstances where phone consultations are necessary. However, you will never know when the information your practised eye gives you will be essential to a successful outcome.

The traditional methods of prescribing for children rely on active observing and perceptive case taking. These skills are universal for all homeopaths, whatever methods they use for case taking or analysis of patient cases. The new methods that will be described in later chapters rely even more on practiced skills in perceiving and understanding what we observe and what this means for the health of the child.

Acute and chronic disease

Many homeopaths view disease and treatment in both adults and children in terms of two major categories: constitutional or acute. Remedies are also divided into those for either acute conditions or the chronic, constitutional problems. There are other homeopaths who assert there is no such divide. They see the problems that are labelled acute as manifestations of the patient's underlying chronic state. In that case there is no such thing as acute and chronic remedies: there are only patients and remedies. As with many topics where there are strongly held opinions on both sides, the reality lies somewhere between the two. For adults, most febrile illnesses, colds and flus, are manifestations of their underlying constitution. Many homeopaths, including myself, have observed that upwards of 80% of these situations are successfully treated with the patient's constitutional remedy. The situation is different with children. At least half, and maybe even the majority of cases, the child's constitutional remedy will not resolve the problem. Another remedy, specific to the immediately presenting symptoms, will be necessary.

Case 2.2   Keynote prescribing

As an example, I recall a lively, delightful two-year-old girl I had treated since birth. She had always done well with her doses of Calcarea carbonica.

One day her grandfather contracted shingles. His lesions appeared only after she had been near him off and on for several days. She was not immunised and had had several years of successful treatment, so there was a good possibility that her innate resistance would prevent any problems. The parents and I were waiting to see if her own healthy immunity was strong enough to tackle that exposure and prevent her presenting any symptoms. She continued to be happy, playful and enchanting. After two weeks, the mother noticed the presence of a few, very small pinpoint red spots on her chest, legs and back. These faded over the next week. About that time, the mother noticed six small red spots slightly larger than the previous spots. The next day she had developed about 30 more spots scattered over her torso, limbs and face. The oldest ones had become like blisters. Interestingly she continued to have no ill effects from these lesions.

Contrary to the expected 'chicken pox' picture, she had no prodromal symptoms or malaise or fever. She continued to play, sleep and eat normally. The spots she did get were few in number, very small and did not bother her. By the third day, some of the spots had started to fade and disappear.

Considering how mild the episode was with no display of distinguishing symptoms or features on which to change her successful constitutional treatment, Calcarea carbonica 30c was repeated. For the first time, she had no relief from her dose. The next day, there was no improvement. To the contrary, about 40 new spots had developed overnight. She was a little restless in the night, but far from the fussy, miserable state that many children have with chickenpox. She still played, was active and displayed her usual energy and lively personality. The only change in her temperament was to be slightly more impatient than usual.

Choice of remedy

Since it was apparent that her usual remedy did not help her, the question was what to do next? Looking at this child's illness as a distinct 'acute' episode, lead me to another remedy altogether. Dispensing with considering her previous indications for Calcarea, I simply focused directly on the problem at hand. Yet, her symptoms were still very mild and nondescript, lending nothing in particular to choose a remedy. Even the tried and true repertorisation was not helpful.

The rubric

- SKIN: Eruptions: Chickenpox

is a large one and in the absence of other defining characteristics to differentiate the remedies there, it is largely of no benefit.

The method that helped was to approach her armed with the experience and empirical knowledge of past clinical cases. This led me to the use of clinical keynotes. From that standpoint, Antimonium crudum was the remedy of choice. It is almost a specific for chickenpox.

Follow up

Within a few hours of the remedy, the parents noticed that the red spots had started to fade! The next day, the lesions had all been scabbed over and were drying up and disappearing. The child was fully recovered within several days. During the entire episode, the child had only 4 or 5 spots that had the appearance of the usual 'normal' chickenpox. The rest came and went quickly, without irritation, pain or scarring.

The above case is an example of what might appear to be old-fashioned keynote prescribing, hardly the kind of case to include in a book about the newer methods of prescribing for children. Yet, this case does exemplify several important points to be kept firmly in mind while reading the rest of the book. Firstly, the traditional tools and wisdom of our predecessors must not be forgotten or overlooked. They did amazing work and deserve to be acknowledged for their skills, many of which are very useful today. Secondly, their approach was often fundamentally not that much different from what is done today and what is described by Hahnemann in the Organon.[5] Regarding the patient in his totality, they found what was to be cured, perceived what was strange, rare and peculiar and finally, sought the simillimum from our materia medica.

With this in mind, another look at this case would be useful. Perceiving the child as a whole, what was really to be cured? She had no symptoms in her general state. She was energetic, happy, lively and as active as always. She had no fever, malaise, appetite change or other disturbance. Her totality was coalesced, congregated in one outstanding symptom – the skin lesions. That is the only thing that needed to be cured. Everything else was healthy and normal. Far from prescribing in a symptomatic way, this case shows the flexibility that is needed when approaching the totality of symptoms. In this case there was a totality of one.

There is an essential distinction between this situation and others in which there are a host of symptoms but only one is selected and used as a keynote. That is not the totality, but symptomatic prescribing reminiscent of allopathic approach. In that approach, one symptom is selected and the rest ignored, even symptoms that may have value. What I described above included all symptoms as a totality; none were ignored. However, there was only one that qualified as a true symptom.

As the use of new methods in children is elaborated, basic principles should be kept in mind. All truly successful methods in homeopathy rest on that strong and solid foundation.

References

1   Borland DM Children's Types (2nd edn) Glasgow: British Homeopathic Association Book Service, 1997.

2   Bryce J 100 Education Quotations compiled by J Pommerville. Available online at http://tinyurl.com/yeqs5pn (Accessed 17th December 2009)

3   Reynolds J Quotes about thoughts and thinking from QuotationsBook.com. Available online at http://tinyurl.com/y8hp39r (Accessed 17th December 2009)

4   Kent JT Repertory of the homoeopathic materia medica (3rd edn) Sittingbourne: Homoeopathic Book Service, 1993.

5   Kunzli J, Naude A, Pendelton P. Organon of Medicine of Samuel Hahnemann, translation from German, 6th edition, Los Angeles, CA: J.P. Tarcher Inc., 1982.

3

NEW APPROACHES
TO CHILDREN'S CASES

The time-honoured methods of treating children have yielded hundreds of thousands of successful results over many decades. Despite these tools, there also have been children for whom these methods have not yielded the healthy outcomes expected. When the limits of any method are reached, it is time to expand our possibilities and explore new ideas. Generally, this is the process by which new techniques of homeopathic practice have been developed, refined and utilised.

Source-based prescribing

The new methods in homeopathy discussed in this book are the techniques developed and explored by Drs. Rajan Sankaran, Jayesh Shah, Divya Chhabra and Sunil Anand,[1] collectively they are termed **source-based** prescribing.

Naturally, any new techniques added to our inventory must be based on first principles. The foundation of homeopathy stays the same; a solid foundation of philosophical and reasoned understanding based on sound biologic, organic and observable reality as expressed in the *Organon of Medicine*.[2] Although these ideas and techniques are called 'new', it is equally accurate to say they are an expansion and elaboration of our traditional approaches, taking the basics of homeopathy to a further extent.

The goal of the homeopath does not change by using the source-based methods. The homeopath still wants to find the simillimum. What is different is the route to get there. How to gather information from the patient, what constitutes the totality of symptoms and recognising the simillimum from those symptoms are a few areas that are different. Most of the techniques of source-based prescribing are based on developing a different set of questions, different criteria for what symptoms are, a different goal for our case taking. What is the child expressing about his worldview by the actions we see and the physical symptoms the child is manifesting? The important skills of observation and interacting with the child are not enough by themselves; the homeopath must understand the significance of what is being observed and what all this information reveals about the source.

A familiarity with the fundamental concepts and techniques of source-based prescribing is necessary to understand how to use them for treating children. The best descriptions can be found in any one of Rajan Sankaran's books, particularly *The Sensation in Homeopathy*[3] and *Sensation Refined*,[4] and the reader is referred to these references for a thorough background in these ideas and any other ideas of Dr. Sankaran's to which this book refers. The basic premises and techniques of source-based prescribing will be discussed, along with other new ideas, especially as they apply to the treatment of children.

Expanding horizons

One of the most exciting and useful aspects of the new ideas and methods in homeopathy is the effect these have had on our materia medica. The great appeal of source-based prescribing is that there is access to remedies that otherwise would never have been used because the traditional sources of information did not provide any data. Even the remedies for which there is information available, it is often of such a general kind as to be virtually useless and would never have been enough to bring that remedy to the forefront on its own. Many times there is no other way to find a remedy than using the new methods because there are no rubrics or materia medica or provings to support the prescription.

Traditionally, the sources of the homeopathic materia medica have included provings, cured cases, herbal information and poisonings. Homeopaths have always regarded provings as the most solidly reliable source of information; the gold standard, the foundation of homeopathy. A good, dependable proving takes some effort and time to accomplish. Hahnemann proved about 100 remedies. Hering proved about 60 between 1820 and 1880. There were very few serious provings for the next 50 years when Drs. Mezger in Germany, Julian and Souk-Aloun in France and Raeside in England together proved about 50 remedies over the next few decades.

With the advent of the new thoughts and directions of homeopathy, there has been a resurgence of interest in provings. Since 1980 many excellent provings have been performed by Jeremy Sherr, Rajan Sankaran, Divya Chhabra, Misha Norland, Jayesh Shah, Todd Rowe, Melanie Grimes, David Riley, Bernd Schuster, Nuala Eising, Uta Santos, Anne Schadde, Karl-Josef Müller, Peter König, Louis Klein, Chetna Shukla, Jonathan Shore and others. This group has added to the materia medica or enlarged the understanding of about 150 remedies, some of which are current mainstays of practice.

Yet, despite all this work, actual provings account for only about 400 remedies. This is a long way from the estimated 3000 remedies mentioned in various materia medicas and the homeopathic literature. The breach has been filled by other sources of information. Even taking into consideration all sources of reliable, trustworthy information, the palette of 3000 remedies is only a faint glimmer compared to the possibilities from the incalculable array of life forms, plants, chemicals and animals available. Working within these confines has been a serious limitation of the traditional methods and ideas.

Case 3.1 Treating asthma

I recall a case I had of a woman with asthma. I tried for four years to find a good remedy for her. Several remedies gave a little relief but most did not affect her at all. I did retake after retake, always trying to find that clue or opening to the case that would point to her simillimum. It was all to no avail; her correct remedy eluded me.

Choice of remedy
The solution was finally found. I was attending a conference by Jeremy Sherr when he discussed the findings of his newly proved remedy, Chocolate.[5] His description of the remedy, the symptoms from a few cured cases and the provings symptoms matched my case perfectly. Thereafter, my patient did exceedingly well on Chocolate for many years.

Many times, I have reflected on this case and its solution. Without the new remedy, Chocolate, she could not have been helped. Although over the years prior to that remedy, she has some degree of improvement, it was far short of what can be achieved with homeopathy and the simillimum. Since that case, whenever I have had a patient whose case seems to elude my best efforts, I would wonder what unproved, undocumented, untried remedy might be what I am seeking. Which out of the millions of possible remedy sources might be right? Then I would turn back to the list of 3000 remedies and try to do my best. Sometimes I felt as if I was trying to write *War and Peace* with two consonants and a vowel.

Source-based prescribing changed all that. It opens up the remedy choices to include every possible substance. In a flash, the materia medica goes from 3000 to millions. It is astonishing how much more accurate, precise and specifically individual prescribing becomes.

The source

Each homeopathic remedy is made from a particular substance, known as its source. The substance as it is known is the physical representation and embodiment of its energy field. It is this energy field that is used in healing with homeopathy. Homeopathy's unique process of potentisation through dilution and succussion essentially releases the energy field from its physical embodiment, thereby activating it for dynamic healing.

Similarly, each person has a unique energy field and he, in his entirety, is the embodiment of that energy field – his source. His individual energy field or source determines his specific 'state of being'. In a state of ideal, perfect health, that field is composed only of the energy of a human being. Perfect health, however, is rarely the case. Most often that energy field is adulterated with another energy. In illness, a particular energy has intertwined itself into the patient's own normal and healthy energy field. The foreign energy exerts influence on the function and expression of a person, altering his healthy state and creating illness. In that circumstance, the human organism, with all its physical, emotional and mental facets, will be directed to display qualities, activities, behaviour, thoughts and body functions that a human being is not designed to do. These 'not human' aspects are experienced as symptoms. Since that energy is an interloper, a foreign visitor, to the human being's energy, it is experienced as unfamiliar and uncomfortable as well as weird, odd and completely irrational. The human organism has several kinds of reactions to this situation, including compensation, hiding, avoidance, suppression or denial of symptoms. All the symptoms and reactions constitute the symptom picture; the reflection of the unknown, interfering energy.

Source-based prescribing

Source-based prescribing entails perceiving the exact nature of this foreign energy; it is the source of the remedy the patient requires. The totality of the 'not-self' expressions constitutes the influence of the 'not-self' energy. The homeopath distinguishes the precise array of these symptoms to ascertain which specific energy has infiltrated the person's normal energy field. What is not part of a person's normal expression of life? The answer to that question identifies the characteristics of the interloping energy. It is known that energy in the form of a remedy is needed for cure. These are basic tenets of homeopathy. Even more than traditional methods, source-based prescribing takes this concept from a philosophic possibility and turns it into practice.

Source-based prescribing rests on the same foundation of homeopathic philosophy that all methods of prescribing do. On one hand, we are required to do as we have always done – find the simillimum from the totality of symptoms. On the other hand, we are doing something new since we are specifically looking for the qualities of the substance's source expressing itself and differentiating those from the person's normal, healthy state.

To accomplish this, several aspects of traditional methods are emphasised, including regarding the whole person in their entirety, looking for the strange, rare and peculiar symptoms as the entry point into the case and incorporating aetiology and susceptibilities (see below). Other areas less explored traditionally that are very fruitful when using source-based methods are dreams, imagination, drawings, parent's life and symptoms, pre-natal experiences and influences as well as the fantasy, playful world of the child. These areas will be explained in full detail in later sections, especially chapter four and the case examples.

The unprejudiced, discriminating perceiver

Case taking

Case taking and prescribing start with the homeopath knowing where his destination is. Where is he headed? Homeopaths know that the goal of treatment is to find the right remedy, the most similar, the simillimum. In source-based prescribing the goal is the same, however, it is phrased slightly different. The homeopath is seeking the source energy as exhibited by the totality of symptoms. There is one, distinct energy orchestrating the entire constellation of a patient's symptoms, characteristics and attitudes, called the 'remedy state' or 'source'. Everything perceived about a patient relates to that source, since ultimately it is the source of the patient's disease. Each and every symptom, each strange, rare and peculiar manifestation, and each distinctive quality leads to the same place – the source. The specific route to the source is less important than recognising when he is on that path and when he has reached the source.

Peculiar or unusual symptoms

Hahnemann's aphorism § 153 states[2]

> 'in the quest for the homeopathically specific remedy, the more striking, strange, unusual, peculiar and characteristic signs and symptoms of the case are especially, almost exclusively, the ones to which close attention should be given'

This mandate has profound significance. To designate something as peculiar or strange requires evaluation and judgement. Yet, at the same time aphorism §6 must also be remembered[2], in which the homeopath is called upon to be the 'unprejudiced observer', meaning that he must not carry preconceived ideas into his clinic. Reconciling these two dictates is the essence of good case taking.

The crux of the matter rests on exactly what is meant by 'peculiar' or 'unusual' and how to objectively recognise when a symptom or characteristic qualifies. Based on the understanding that symptoms arise from a human energy field contaminated by a foreign, non-human energy, the homeopath defines 'strange, peculiar and unusual' as those symptoms that are from that alien source. Perceiving what is not the usual human behaviour, reaction or quality is to open the door to perceiving the source energy disrupting normal human health. It is his task, therefore, to be able to distinguish the normal from the not normal, the usual from the not usual, the expected from the not expected; in short, to distinguish what is human from not human. Yes, he must judge and discriminate. How can the homeopath do that in a neutral, unprejudiced way?

The importance of discrimination

The trend in recent decades has been to disparage the act of discriminating. People are admonished, even legally constrained, from discriminating and being prejudiced. The two are actually very different acts. To discriminate is to recognise the differences between two things, which is simply to distinguish between qualities, designating one as good or normal and the other not. That is a natural and automatic analytic function, without which we could not survive. Prejudice is to have a preformed opinion not based on sufficient knowledge, reason or actual experience. Though typically thought to be always a bad thing to do, this ability too is an important function. Everyone draws on second-hand experiences and insufficient information in making choices and conclusions. It is functionally and neurologically impossible not to. If the homeopath is consciously aware of this tendency, he will be more likely to follow Hahnemann's warning and refrain from allowing any preconceived ideas from interfering with the open-minded process of perceiving what the patient is telling him. By doing so, it is possible to properly discriminate the normal and expected from the strange, unusual and peculiar. The homeopath becomes an unprejudiced, discriminating perceiver.

Normal and not normal

The biggest assistance in making these critical distinctions in a useful way is to be fully aware of what is normal, usual and expected. This is complicated because what is considered normal changes. Throughout a person's entire life, there are transitions, transformations and stages, each with its own normalcy. Understanding what, when and at what stage behaviour is normal is decisively important. Each stage of development is normal at its correct time and place, and in the right sequence. What is appropriate for a teen is not expected in a 40 year old. What is normal at 40 is far from healthy in a child. For example, everyone has had the experience of being totally dependent on their mother for their very life. The right time and place for that experience were the months of intrauterine life. If someone is still experiencing that level of helpless dependency at age 5 or 15 or 50, it is not normal. Getting stuck or stopping at a particular point of development constitutes pathology.

Understanding how a child's neurological system and brain develop, their relationship to his unfolding behaviour, mental advancement and acquisition of skills allows the homeopath to see clearly what is not going according to the normal plan. The changes in childhood are more rapid, extensive and fundamental than at any other time of life. So swift are the transitions that what is expected for a 12 month old, is not normal for either a six month or 18 month old. Chapter four contains enough detail about normal childhood development to assist making these crucial assessments. It cannot be stressed enough how important it is for the homeopath to have a thorough familiarity with the physical, emotional, and mental stages of child development. This knowledge is akin to the pianist learning scales or the artist mixing color tints. It is the necessary foundation on which all observation and perceptions about the child will rest.

Being stuck

In the example above, the energy of that stage of helpless dependency is stable and present during foetal life. That energy is also present in the world at large in various forms, each with its own distinctive nuances of expression. Plants, minerals, animals, microorganisms and other life forms and substances are each the expression of one specific energy on earth. When someone experiences this stage other than at the right time, energy is needed in one of the other earthly forms to allow development to continue. Stuck in the helplessly dependent, umbilical stage of life results in symptoms, requiring that exact missing energy to emerge from it.

The question for the homeopath is – which energy is it?

Homeopaths do not prescribe based on the situation, but rather on the energy source as evidenced by the manifestation of that exact array of symptoms experienced by the patient. The key is the way the patients perceive and experiences their life and 'stuckness'.

In the example, the patient may perceive it as a curtailing of structural development requiring the energy of Lithium or as a block to growth needing a Euphorbiaceae's energy or as a problem with attachment needing one of the Malvaceae's energies. The source energy of each of these three different substances will result in a subtly different experience for the patient. Source-based prescribing necessitates that we reach that level of the patient's experience to perceive these differences and not settle for a superficial aetiology, situation or single symptom.

Getting stuck at a stage occurs when a specific life function has not developed. The often used rubric,

- GENERALITIES: Development arrested

is woefully deficient because all illness is arrested development in one form or another; staying stuck at some stage of development and preceding no further. A challenge has not been overcome, a function has not developed, and an aspect of being a fully free functioning human being is delayed, missing or incomplete.

One consequence is that what should have been done automatically must be done manually or consciously. Experiencing anticipation anxiety is often the signal that a usually automatic function has to be done consciously with attention and intention. The stage of development provides less capability or functionality than the situation requires. For example, breathing is an automatic action. What anxiety a person would experience if it was necessary to consciously remember to breathe! He would not be able to do anything else such as think, analyse or create because every few seconds he would have to remember to work those lungs.

Likewise, appetite and hunger are automatic functions. Reflect for a moment on how much time and effort people consciously spend managing their appetite, food choices, calorie intake, nutrient levels and other dietary issues. All of this work is done manually for functions that are designed to be automatic. In a state of real health, hunger and appetite are balanced, accurate and properly functioning for optimum body performance without any conscious effort. All the attention and effort is then available for more creative and interesting pursuits.

Inner conflict

All life has an innate drive towards expression, growth and exploration. Every advance necessitates leaving a state of stability and familiarity, thus initiating challenge and risk. Despite the often felt desire to hold on to what is successful and familiar, in nature there is no possibility of staying static, resting on one's laurels content with the status quo. There is either forward movement or decline.

In health, there is enough energy and confidence to forge ahead to face whatever challenge presents itself. In illness, however, attachment to the known is in conflict with the drive for growth. The normal developmental desire to move forward and explore is overcome by the fear of losing the bond to the safe place of familiarity, yet staying put leads to stagnation and arrested development. Either way, having these two opposing drives results in illness and symptoms.

If the sick child tries to follow his drive for exploration, he feels unsafe and insecure triggering fear and anxiety, which serves to stop his forward growth. If he stays secure in his familiar surroundings, his fear is gone, but he will be frustrated and irritated at the inability of his forward drive to be expressed. There is no way out, no resolution. Illness always puts a person in this kind of no-win, double-bind position. Neither option gives the unalloyed benefit of normal development. Each provides only a hint of relief mixed with a large dose of disadvantage. Divya Chhabra calls these the classic Catch-22 situations, a phrase coined by author Joseph Heller from his 1961 book of that name.[6] Now in general usage, the term signifies a situation of endless circular argument of conflicting considerations, without any solution.

Whenever the child has symptoms, we know that his natural, innate drive to grow has been thwarted. There is some countervailing force stopping that drive, creating the double-bind, Catch-22 situation. To understand, we must ask what two opposing forces are in conflict, thereby making the child stuck and unable to move forward in life. On one side is his stage of development and the other will be the specific sensation or feeling hindering him.

Each remedy's energy encompasses one particular kind of Catch-22 dilemma. For a specific example, consider Natrum muriaticum. On one side, a person requiring Natrum mur. feels irresistibly driven to attach closely and intimately to one other person, even to the point of entwining his identity with the other's. If that were the only driving force, there would be no conflict. The person would find an intimate partner and stay attached. The opposing drive creates the dilemma. Natrum mur. also has the strong element of feeling abject disappointment at having their expectations unfulfilled, resulting in a wary withdraw into self-reliance and bitterness. The Catch-22 of Natrum mur. is feeling drawn to form a tight, close bond with one other but if he does, he will inevitably be disappointed and deeply hurt by that person. If he protects himself from any hurt by staying alone and self-sufficient, walled off from relationships, he feels completely lonely and unfulfilled, restlessly driven to attach to that special someone. The circle completes as their drive to become attached propels them to form a close, intimate bond, thereby, once again exposing them to potential disappointment and hurt. Around it goes, a never-ending dilemma with no way out. Only the remedy can break the cycle and release the person to be able to form healthy relationships.

In some of the ensuing case examples, the stuck point or Catch-22 will be highlighted in order to see how this idea is expressed in patients.

Sankaran and miasms

One of the most insightful and helpful developments in homeopathy has been Dr. Rajan Sankaran's explanation and use of miasms in prescribing.[7] A full treatment of this fascinating subject is beyond the scope of this book but the following few comments will serve as an introduction to his ideas.

Dr. Sankaran sees a miasm as the 'depth of the disease', meaning how seriously and deeply has the illness affected the patient; how desperate has the illness made the patient. There are ten miasms, arranged in order of increasing severity and desperation, each with its own identifying description. This construct assists in prescribing, by giving the homeopath another perspective from which to understand the patient. Where I have found these ideas the most beneficial is in understanding and using the plant kingdom remedies.

Thanks to such innovative thinkers as Drs. Sankaran, Jayesh Shah and Diyva Chhabra, homeopathy has progressed to the understanding that groups of remedies in the same zoological, botanical or chemical groups have many similar symptoms and characteristics. Group or family themes have been of enormous benefit in finding a correct remedy and utilising previously little known remedies to great effect. Their elucidation of the themes and sensations for the many plant families and groupings has opened up a world of plant remedies that hitherto had been neglected. With plants, however, knowing the family themes and sensations was not enough. With so many remedies in each family exhibiting the same family themes, how was it possible to differentiate among them? The answer is the use of the miasms concept. Each plant within a single botanical grouping displays the characteristics of one of the ten miasms. Identifying the family through the patient's sensation combined with the miasm from the level of desperation in the patient's reactions delineates the remedy required.

My thumbnail description hardly does justice to the sophistication, elegance and usefulness of these ideas. Many homeopaths have found them exceedingly helpful. In the following pages, there are case examples that utilise this system of family themes and miasms. From then it will be possible to see this system in action.

The compensated patient

As a person goes about his life, living an energy state infused with a foreign energy, he exhibits those characteristics, thoughts and actions. This is the involuntary process of having a symptom producing disease. Naturally, a person does not like to have symptoms. At best, they are annoying and at worst, they can be debilitating or life threatening. Additionally, many emotional or mental symptoms can be dangerous, cause legal problems or are disruptive to social and civilised living. It is one thing for a person to be in his state, living out the dictates of the energy force inside him and it is another thing entirely to be able to be effective in life and function in society with the specific array of characteristics and symptoms. Even a terse glance through a repertory's mind section gives an idea of what havoc there would be if people gave free reign to the pure inner state of disease.

From an early age, people disguise the less appealing, disruptive and unworkable symptoms, the ones that are just not practicable or feasible to display. Some symptoms are consciously avoided, altered or suppressed. Many others are hidden as a result of the action of the body's own inner defence and are quite involuntary. The end result is that symptoms are concealed, camouflaged, altered and suppressed, all classified as compensation. Often a significant portion of case taking is taken up simply with getting underneath these various alterations and suppressions to be able to perceive the real symptoms and uncompensated state, which is necessary to prescribe correctly.

Overall children live in a far less compensated state, thereby experiencing their authentic state without the overlay of suppressions and alterations. This is great news for the homeopath. In most children's cases what the homeopath sees is what he gets; the symptoms are clear and the state is directly expressed.

For example, a Stramonium child vociferously and unabashedly expresses his fear of the dark, fear of monsters under the bed, fear of people chasing after him and his desire to cling to his mother. He may even hit or be aggressive with other children without reservation. An adult Stramonium, having been socialised and having learned that he cannot successfully function displaying those traits, will not act that way. He most certainly still has those feelings and inclinations, but now they are expressed in an altered, suppressed or disguised way. The fears and aggression are evident in either physical symptoms or some socially acceptable format such as in hobbies, movies or sports. Without looking deeply into the life of the adult Stramonium patient, the homeopath may not see the indications for the remedy. The child is far more likely to still be expressing symptoms in their pure form. They are living closer to the source and its expressions. That makes our job just that much easier.

Where is the energy?

In addition to their energy state, people have a resource of vitality, called vital energy, used to live, grow, develop, cope and function. In a state of health, there is enough vital energy to perform all the tasks needed to maintain and continue development of the person at whatever stage of life they are living. Symptoms occur when there is a deficit of vital energy; the demands of living outpace the person's supply. Some symptoms originate from the organism's efforts at conserving its limited supply of vital energy by eliminating certain activities. Growth is among the areas that slow down or stop when there is not enough vital energy available. It can be regarded that the remedy is either a source of this vital energy or removes the blocks to the organism from utilising its own. Either way, after a dose of the correct remedy, the organism will have enough energy to restore all functions to normal, including growth and maturation.

Specific events during the process of maturation and development can be the source of the deficiency of vital energy. Bone growth, mental development, learning, teething, social adjustments, puberty, skill acquisition and many other aspects of normal childhood all require vital energy, and often require more than is available.

Frequently a child's cold, flu or ear infection will be the reason that the mother brings the child to your clinic. After the remedy, as expected, the child improves; the cold and ear problem is gone. The next day, however a tooth erupts that had been sequestered below the gum line, all the while seeming to be progressing normally. In actuality, forming that tooth and pushing it to the surface had taken so much energy that the organism had run out before completing the job. Hence, dentition stalled. Once the vital energy supply was deficient, other symptoms occurred in the form of a cold or ear infection.

Children do not simply become sick. They display symptoms when their energy is deficient to do the job at hand. This perspective is extremely helpful in treating children. Approaching the child knowing what the normal tasks are at any given age, and then enquiring into where the child's vital energy has gone to create such a deficiency will yield very useful information to help the child.

What to expect?

The following chapters will further discuss the basic principles, techniques and methods of source-based prescribing and other new ideas in homeopathy. Additionally, there will be cases to exemplify these and other key points. The result of all of this is, of course, being able to prescribe the curative remedy and manage the patient case to achieve maximum benefit. The general focus is on case taking and prescribing. What about the results of treatment? What should be expected with the right remedy?

By using these new methods rather than some of the more traditional ones, our goals are commensurate with these perspectives. Given that disease is being stuck in a stage of growth or in an unresolved dilemma, healing is to recommence growth and rise out of the dilemma. How does that look in the patient? Naturally it is expected that all the symptoms resolve. Additionally, in children, after the correct remedy there is a surge of growth. I have seen children gain centimeters in height and kilograms in weight in a matter of weeks. Mental development also exhibits its own leap forward, as the rate of learning gains speed. Maturation on all levels blossoms, making up for lost time caused by the constraints of illness. Teeth erupt, clothing becomes too tight and trousers suddenly are too short, new interests emerge, confidence is displayed, fears evaporate and happiness is restored. Free of illness, the child can fully enjoy the kaleidoscope of adventures that childhood offers.

Knowing normal

From the discussion so far, it must be clear that in order to successfully under-stand symptoms and illness, there must be a thorough understanding of the normal stages of child development in all aspects; the physical, emotional and mental. Any stress, problem or dilemma a child has will be in the context of their normal changes and growth. What is normal and expected must be taken into consideration to be able to see the contrast of what might be signs of a problem such as a reaction out of place or too extreme, the absence of a normal response and the opposing drives of a Catch-22 dilemma.

Before going any further in describing case taking, source-based prescribing or other aspects of methodology, it will be of inestimable value to take the time to elaborate in detail about normal childhood development and the special characteristics of childhood encountered and relevant to childhood treatment. This foundation, provided in chapter four, will allow the homeopath more easily to perceive what is going wrong with the normal, healthy unfolding of the child's natural growth and development. Additionally, this information will greatly serve to understand and utilise the source-based prescribing techniques more successfully.

References

1   Author's personal notes 1996-2009.
2   Kunzli J, Naude A, Pendelton P. Organon of Medicine of Samuel Hahnemann, translation from German, 6th edition, Los Angeles, CA: J.P. Tarcher Inc., 1982.
3   Sankaran R. The Sensation in Homeopathy. Mumbai: Homeopathic Medical Publishers, 2004.

4   Sankaran R. Sensation Refined. Mumbai: Homeopathic Medical Publishers, 2007.
5   Sherr J. The homoeopathic proving of chocolate. Worcester: Dynamis, 1993.
6   Heller J. Catch-22 New York, NY: Simon and Schuster, 1961.
7   Author's personal notes from seminars 2000–2009.

4

CHILDHOOD DEVELOPMENT

PART ONE – A SPECIAL TIME OF LIFE

The treatment of children has its distinctive challenges and requires something above and beyond how we approach adults. Childhood is special and demands something special from us. Before attempting to treat children, we should understand what childhood is and what happens to the child during these important years.

What exactly is childhood?

Is it simply a range of ages? Is it a stage delineated by specific growth and development? What is unique about these years? What characterises childhood to make this time of life special and so challenging?

One of the first distinctive characteristics about childhood is that it lasts so long compared to other mammals. As a group, humans have far more capacity, versatility, educability, creativity and flexibility than any other animal. Our increased prowess requires more time for preparation to bring our potential into fruition. As a result, humans have a longer period of dependence, or childhood, than any other species. Childhood comprises an amazing series of stages of development over about 14 years.

Never again in life will there be such growth as there is in childhood. By the end of the first year of life, the child weighs three times as much as at birth. By age two, the brain has tripled in weight. During the first few years, a child gains an average of about 25 cm (10 in) in height each year. Even puberty, with its famed growth spurt, only achieves a maximum of about 10 cm (4 in) per year. Growth is not just in physical size; mental development, language skills and all manner of learning advance with astounding speed. In four scant years the child is transformed from being a totally dependent newborn who is unable to regulate body temperature or focus the eyes to being a verbal, ambulatory, inquisitive, mechanically adept, social individual. Of course, even at this age, the infant child is still dependent and will be so for many years to come but the changes have been dramatic.

All of this growth and development requires energy. This does not simply refer to adequate food and nutrients. Enough vital energy, or life force, is required. Under ideal conditions the child has all the energy needed for the process of birth, growth, development and living. When there is not enough energy to fuel these natural processes, they slow down or stop and symptoms develop. Childhood illnesses occur when there is a discrepancy between the energy required for growth and the amount available. The causes of an energy shortage have been mentioned in chapter three and will be discussed in later chapters. For now, it is sufficient to say an energy deficit results in specific symptoms, which tell the homeopath exactly where the problem lies. It is his or her job to identify the developmental processes that have stopped and find the right remedy to restore the child's vitality so that health and growth can be recommenced.

A child's miraculous unfolding is orchestrated with awesome perfection. Conception, the experiences in the nine months of intrauterine life, through birth, the first moments after birth and the childhood years all play critical roles in determining what will follow. If any step along this precise cascade of sequential stages is missed, it will upset or delay every single step further down the path. To a large degree these years lay the foundation for health or susceptibility to illness, what kind of symptoms may develop and how a child will experience the entire rest of his life: health or illness, happiness or misery, ease or anxiety. Every homeopath has seen adults whose entire life experience has been shaped from the lack of some important mental or emotional development from childhood. With so much indispensable formative development taking place, true full health in childhood is critically important.

There are many excellent and readily available books on childhood developmental stages. It is not the intention to repeat here what others have described so effectively. However, certain key points and principles that have direct bearing on the homeopathic treatment of children will be discussed.

Child development

When investigating child development, including the physical, mental and emotional aspects of childhood, there is something important to keep in mind. Most of the existing books written, research performed or ideas accepted are based on observations on what are regarded as 'normal' children or what are taken as 'normal' expectations of childhood. These are children whom homeopaths might regard as unhealthy to some degree. The conventional world has no notion of a fully functional healthy state because all their models are dysfunctional. When a malady becomes the rule rather than the exception, or when its presence is widespread, then the dysfunction is accepted as a normal condition.

For example, among most parents it is accepted as normal that pre-school aged children may have from one to five ear infections per year, or experience numerous colds and episodes of congestion. Parents and teachers expect that when children first start school, they will become unwell more often. Tantrums are thought to be normal for two-year-olds. How many parents wait with anxiety and trepidation for the time when their child reaches puberty because it is common knowledge that the teen years are fraught with hostility, rebellion and difficulty? There are many more examples of conditions accepted by the conventional world as normal, whereas in fact these situations are evidence of ill health, or as homeopaths would say, a deficit of vital energy. These symptoms that are widely accepted as inescapable aspects of growing, improve with homeopathic treatment, thereby verifying that they are aspects of illness.

Homeopaths regard pre-natal life, newborns, infants and children by different standards than most others. They do not accept the levels of ill health and symptoms that are so commonly classified as normal and therefore must be tolerated. Remember to keep this in mind while referring to anything written from the allopathic perspective. For those who treat children with homeopathy, it is possible to witness the wonder and miraculous joy of a child growing and evolving in a state of health.

Continual development

Human development is a continuum from the moment of conception throughout our entire life, possibly beyond. Each stage in life is built from and depends upon all that has come before. Nature has orchestrated our continuum of development in an awe-inspiring and complete way. We have everything we need to be born, grow and flourish, being able, as Hahnemann says in the Organon 'to freely use this living, healthy instrument for the higher purposes of our existence.'[1]

For the complete unfurling of human potential, a person experiences repeated cycles of growth and development throughout his entire life. This cyclic pattern requires three main components: stability, possibilities and energy. A stable, safe environment is required, plus the urge to extend beyond that immediate safe place to explore unknown possibilities plus the energy, resources and confidence with which to accomplish it. The process starts by establishing a stable ground of familiarity from which to launch growth into the mysterious and unexplored. As a person explores, he incorporates the previously mystifying into a broader place of familiar ground. From that new and larger base, he can again venture into the unknown for further exploration and experiences. In health, this kind of growth pattern continues throughout a person's entire life, with each stage of life being an extension and expansion of himself into a larger, more varied, more encompassing world.

The American philosopher Mortimer Adler (1902–2001) observed,

> 'The purpose of learning is growth, and our minds, unlike our bodies, can continue growing as long as we live.'[2]

Here is health in its most fundamental sense; the freedom for a person to become all he can be and to realise his full potential as a human being.

This cyclic developmental pattern occurs many times throughout childhood. Becoming familiar with each component will greatly help achieve understanding on how and why a child becomes ill. It is possible to determine in which age or stage a child is by what he is willing and is unwilling to explore. Understanding starts by investigating each aspect of this process. A person will start with a safe, familiar place that gives comfort and security. Safe is not the most accurate word. Life itself is never completely safe. By its very nature, being alive means being exposed to risks, challenges, hazards, possibilities and unrealised or thwarted potentials. A person is perpetually encountering risky situations; some of great risk, others of low risk. In practical terms, the idea of safe means an environment of relatively low risk. A person will feel at home and this familiarity gives him security, ease and confidence. Safety even encompasses identity as the experience of his own inner strength and capacities supports his sense of identity. He knows who he is and what he can do.

As comfortable and confident as a person feels in a familiar safe place, there is also an innate drive to look outward beyond, to expand and reach for what is beyond the grasp. What's out there? All human development, the advance of civilisation, all progress, invention and discovery has sprung from man's inherent drive to know. What else is outside the bounds of safety? Out beyond are opportunities, challenges, potential and objects of curiosity. Development and growth depend on these possibilities. There is somewhere to go. There is a beckoning destination; the intriguing unknown whetting the appetite for exploration, to find out, to learn. The low risk, safe place, affords a person the stability and confidence from which he can venture into challenges of higher risk, thereby transforming himself into a more fully developed person.

The final ingredient to the triad is energy; the emotional, physical and spiritual power and resources to fuel the movement from safety to challenge. If there is ever any doubt about this drive being a fundamental part of all life, there is evidence of it all around. Even the commonplace reveals this compelling drive. Sprigs of plants grow up through the tiny cracks in a concrete slab. Imagine the vigour and force that obliges the seedling to take on the challenge of growing through concrete. Miraculously it winds its way though a microscopic crevice so it can burst through to the sunlit sky. Acting on the stability of the seed, enough force allows the growing plant to embrace the challenge of living, eventually pushing aside the concrete.

All people go through this cycle in a continual process of resting with confidence in a safe place, looking beyond to greater possibilities and then gathering the energy and resources to venture forth to meet a new challenge. Finally, the new knowledge and strength is incorporated into the ever-expanding self thus establishing a new safe place on a wider plateau. This template of development is seen many times over in the growing child in a variety of situations and challenges.

American psychologist Abraham Maslow (1908-1970) said,

> 'All the evidence that we have indicates that it is reasonable to assume in practically every human being, and certainly in almost every newborn baby, that there is an active will toward health, an impulse towards growth, or towards the actualisation.'[3]

In this and later chapters, the details of this process as it applies to children will be elaborated, showing how important this understanding is to successful treatment.

A person goes from womb to mother to family to community to the world, each stage providing increasing possibilities for reaching the higher purposes of human existence. Many homeopaths have understood that these stages and the developmental challenges they bring, are represented by the elements and the periodic table. Life's progress is revealed from the energy of conception in hydrogen to the return to the quantum energy from which it started, as demonstrated by the overtly physical deterioration of the radioactive elements beyond radon. Each element in between concretises a particular challenge and experience of human growth and development. The array of elements traverses the progressive stages in the same order that a person does. Each stage must be mastered before expanding into the next. A person masters a challenge by facing it with energy, intention and desire until this new arena becomes familiar and safe again. Once safe, he can turn his life force to another challenge, and so goes the process of life and living.

Obviously this is not to say that all people require remedies from the mineral kingdom. Far from it: homeopathy derives remedies from plants, animals, microorganisms, fungi and imponderables. Irrespective of the kind of remedy a person requires, the periodic table's arrangement of the elements teaches a great deal about the normal, expected stages of development, especially about children's growth. This process and the periodic table will be considered as an example of the stages of growth and development throughout the book. Understanding what is normal is critical to be able to identify what is not healthy and therefore requires improvement.

To everything there is a season

Benjamin Franklin (1706–1790) observed in a letter to the French physicist Jean-Baptiste Leroy, on 13th November 1789,

'In this world nothing can be said to be certain except death and taxes.'[4]

One more item may be added to that list of certainties: Nature programmes for success. The stages, goals, needs, imperatives and progress designed to occur in childhood are part of that plan for success. Each child has an innate desire for growth, a life force from within driving him forward in progress and development. This allows, actually compels, the child to flourish. The child's mind, emotions and physical body are distinctly endowed with the abilities to meet the particular challenges of his growth and development.

Consider a few examples. During this time of life a child learns to walk. There is a very specific moment in the overall scheme of the myriad aspects of development that walking must take place. Many things are happening at the same time in the growing child. There is physical growth of every part of his body – bones, muscles, digestion, brain and nervous system. Concomitant with brain growth is an explosion of learning, along with zestful curiosity to explore the surrounding world.

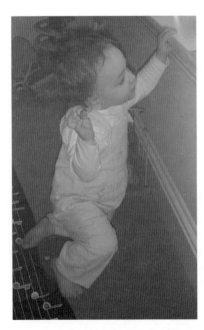

Figure 4.1 When the child has sufficient muscle strength he pulls himself up.

There comes a moment when the child is saturated with the learning his immediate surroundings can offer. His gaze, mental and physical, looks past his reach. What is out there?

Physical development

Standing   Safe and confident enough with the stability of where he is, the child yearns to venture forth and he does. As it happens, this occurs exactly at the time when the child's body weight is light enough for the developing muscles in his arms to have the strength to pull himself up by grasping a table edge (see figure 4.1).

Once up, his legs are just strong enough to keep him up. While the child is standing holding the table, his leg muscles strengthen (see figure 4.2). Standing

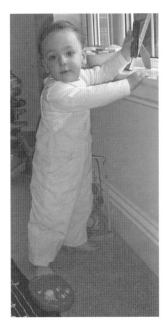

Figure 4.2 While the child is standing and holding on the leg muscles strengthen.

upright supported by the table – or a parent – allows the neurological circuitry of balance and movement to be refined for full functioning (see figure 4.3).

After some days of these calisthenics his leg strength and balance increase to the point where he will no longer need the prop. Feeling secure, the previously unfamiliar world of standing and holding onto the table is now familiar territory. He can do what he could not do just days before. That mastered, he is ready to

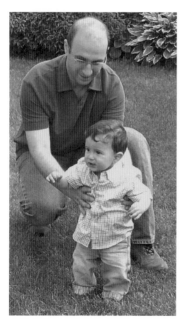

Figure 4.3 Support is also given by a parent.

try something else new. Letting go, the child stands on his own. Success! But what's next? The beyond is still beckoning, motivating those first steps to be taken. Initially faltering, feeble and falling, then courageous, convinced and confident, the child walks.

Walking   All the child's systems and development converge for the accomplishment of this task at hand, each playing its crucial part in the success. What might happen if this precise timetable is disrupted? The interference might be something as minor as the child being carried about by the parent too long, or more serious circumstances such as the bones being weak from malnutrition or the environment being so impoverished or frightening that there is no chance for independent movement. The complexity of development lends itself to many possible problems. For whatever reason, if the window of opportunity for the child to pull himself up and stand supported is missed, then he will not learn to walk so easily. At the precise moment that the child has the innate urge to walk, his body is exactly the right weight for his muscle mass and strength to be able to pull and hold him up (see figure 4.4).

Should that manoeuvre be delayed, the child's body will continue to grow, very rapidly becoming too heavy for his small and now unpractised muscles to lift him up. If he cannot pull himself up with his arms to stand supported by the table, his leg muscles will not get the workout they need to strengthen. Without

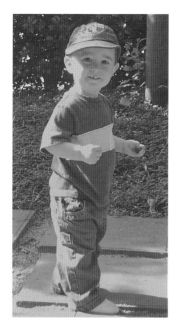

Figure 4.4 At the precise moment that the child has the innate urge to walk, his body is exactly the right weight.

leg strength, walking won't take place. Even if the urge to walk is still there because the mental development is on target, the delay in the physical time frame will disrupt the overall progress.

This window is a very narrow one, and the best development is when the child goes through it at just the right time. This is not to say that a child missing this moment will never walk. Of course he will, but it is much harder to accomplish. Additionally, this missed or delayed milestone launches a cascade of other problems as the whole developmental sequential schedule is upset.

The following rubrics summarise the result, irrespective of what part of the process was disrupted.[5]

- EXTREMITIES; Walk, late learning to,
- EXTREMITIES; Weakness, Lower Limbs, child late learning to walk

Teething   Teething is another milestone of child growth (see figure 4.5). A teething child has the reputation of being extremely fussy or crying inconsolably, often to the chagrin of the whole household.

A few of the usual rubrics used are shown below:

- GENERALITIES; Dentition difficult
- TEETH; Dentition difficult
- MOUTH; Pain; Gums; dentition aggravated

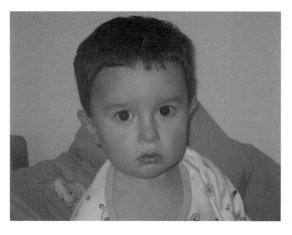

*Figure 4.5 Teething is
a natural stage of
growth but causes
distress and difficulty.*

- MOUTH; Pain; Children, in, during dentition
- MIND; Dentition aggravated
- MIND; Irritability; dentition aggravated
- MIND; Shrieking; Dentition aggravated
- MIND; Weeping; in children from difficult dentition.

Since teething is a natural stage of growth, how can it cause so much distress and difficulty? The answer lies in the orchestrated sequence of healthy growth. Teething is not one event; it is not merely a tooth becoming visible as it pokes its way through the gums. It is a process that starts in the foetus and continues for many years in episodes of more or less activity. Like most body structures, teeth are initially formed during gestation. After birth, they continue to grow below the gums. As the tooth tissue mineralises with calcium, it becomes stronger and larger. Between about four to eight months, some teeth have matured to the point where they are ready to become functional teeth. Slowly, the tooth moves up through the gums, until the first glimpse of its hard, pearly surface is seen in the midst of the soft, pink gums.

It is assumed that this process involves a hard, sharp tooth that cuts its way through the sensitive gums. So ingrained is this idea that the process is usually called 'cutting a tooth.' No wonder the child cries! This is not the whole story. Healthy dentition is painless or nearly so. As some doctors from the 1900s stated, '*dentition is as painless a process as the growing of fingernails.*'[6] It may be hard to believe with the cries of so many distressed teething children still ringing in everyone's ears. Yet, no one has stopped to ask, 'Why wouldn't that be so?' Why wouldn't this natural, expected process of maturation proceed with ease? After all, Nature programmes for success, not distress.

In a healthy child, dentition and all the other developmental activities are taking place at the right time and in the right way. The tooth slowly grows upward through the gum. It does not cut the gums. The pace is just right to allow the tooth to exert pressure against the gum tissue to reduce its blood supply and numb the nerve endings. The continued, gradually increasing pressure causes that tissue to wither or shrink away to the point of allowing the tooth to move through it easily and painlessly. It acts like a snowplough moving through a large snowdrift. To compare to dentition, instead of the vehicle's blade cutting through the snow forcing it aside with effort, imagine that the snow moves aside on its own just as the pressure of the oncoming plough barely touches it. This is an image closer to how the gum tissue is designed to 'move aside' to make way as the tooth approaches. Even the last push through the final gum barrier to reveal its shiny presence should be painless, as the gums have been prepared well ahead of time to expect that eruption. Many children's dentition process is heralded by their increased desire to press their gums onto hard objects, which they do with great relish! If the tooth forging ahead were actually cutting the gums, each chomp would be painful. On the contrary, it affords the child great relief. The child is assisting the tooth in its job of pressing the gum tissue to ensure pain-lessness of the process.

Dentition is painful when this built-in mechanism does not take place at the right time and in the right way. This can occur if the teeth have not developed properly due to inadequate calcium or other nutrients, or from any other obstruction or disturbance to any aspect of the normal pattern of development. If the child's energy and resources are being used in some other area, such as coping with an unusual stressor, fright, illness, disruptive household or other anxiety, then there will not be enough energy to devote to the normal timetable of teething. The sequence has been disorganised and the mechanism by which the gums allow for painless teeth transit, will not be working. Then teething can be extremely painful.

These are just two simple examples of the amazing precision by which growth and development have been designed for maximum ease and progress. When any one of the many steps is delayed, incompletely performed or interrupted, symptoms will arise. In fact, when symptoms are present, you can take that as proof-positive that some aspect of normal progress has been thwarted. Symptoms are our clues that the otherwise smooth path of growth has been strewn with pebbles, or even boulders. Knowing what Nature provides for a child's growth progression, we can see where it has stopped, thus enabling us to smooth the way again.

Mental development

A child's mental, emotional and spiritual growth have developmental timetables just as precise and complex as the physical growth schedule and are just as important to understand. Furthermore, physical, mental and emotional aspects are inseparably intertwined; their developmental stages act synergistically. Muscles cannot advance without the signals from nerves initiating contractions. Those signals come from the maturing brain, which is learning and thinking about new things continuously. Feedback from the world comes back to the brain through sensory input, which then further enhances learning and enacts new motor action. All of this developmental progress is completely intertwined with brain function and growth, which determines the unfolding of mental and emotional stages of development and capacity.

It is easy to overlook this relationship when assessing developmental stages. Neurological development is demonstrated in a child's behaviour, learning and growth. Parents enjoy watching the advent of their child following an object with his eyes and grasping it. The eyes, eye muscles and eye-hand coordination are becoming more functional, all of which are, of course, connected to the brain. The key player in this milestone is brain maturation. The same occurs with sitting up or walking. The physical components of muscle, bone and balance from the inner ear are easy to see in these achievements, yet here too, brain and neurological development is central and primary.

Being able to understand and communicate with children is greatly assisted by having a firm grasp of the process of neurological development to know what their brains are able to do at any given age, and therefore what to expect of the child's progress. The field of brain function and development is enormous; shelves of books have been written on every small aspect. It is far too complex, and actually controversial, to elaborate in too much detail but a few comments are necessary and applicable for this discussion of helping to understand and prescribe for children. Becoming familiar with the neuroanatomy and development involved helps to perceive what kind of learning and growth are taking place and therefore what to expect from children, making it possible to detect what aspect of this process may have been faulty, delayed or missed. The child's mental connection to his body is the basis for how he develops and expresses illness and symptoms. For the homeopath, this perspective can be immensely helpful in selecting the right remedy and planning for the unfolding of the healing process.

Brain growth

The brain does not simply grow; it develops in an intricately orchestrated sequence of steps. If some aspect of the neuron circuitry has not yet blossomed or become serviceable, then it is unrealistic to expect those functions to be performed. Often certain milestones of mental development and skill acquisition are thought to be solely a matter of training or education. Generally, this is not the case. For training to work and learning to take place, the area of the brain related to that neurological function must mature first.

There is heated debate about what is the predominant influence on man's development.

Are we genetically programmed or are we the product of outside influences such as upbringing and environment? Which is more important – nature or nurture? Most now agree that the two are intertwined and interrelated to such a degree that neither is the most important, nor can one do without the other. In harmonious interaction, both determine how we develop. The genetic endowment is the brain's blueprint determining general anatomy and functions, the generic set of qualities. Environmental influences of sensory stimulation and experience refine and extend the network of synaptic connections, thereby acting on the generic to create the specific, unique attributes and capabilities.

Under genetic control, brain formation starts just weeks after conception. Brain cells multiply at the astonishing rate of about 250,000 per minute and begin their migration to the various regions of the brain where they will stay to perform their final functions. Cells also must extend an arm called an axon, to find and connect to other neuron cells and various end organs like muscles, ears, eyes, heart and all others. Many thousands of genes orchestrate this interconnected synaptic network including body end organs. This is the genetic or 'nature' component.

As the nerve forms, gets situated and interconnected, its early activity helps determine what additional activity and connections it will have. A nerve's activity strongly influences its own growth. Stimulation increases the brain's capacity for more stimulation through greater inter-connectability. The number and extent of these connections between neurons and organs is a critical factor in advancing brain development, versatility and function. These external factors play their critical role by their specific quantity and quality, as well as their presence or absence during certain critical periods of development. The result is a perfection of brain development, responsive to the needs as provided to it from external stimulation. This is the environmental or 'nurture' component.

For the most part, the entire brain with its 100 billion neurons is formed by the time of birth and, with rare exception, a person has all he is ever going to have when he is born. Interestingly, the infant brain actually contains substantially more neurons than the adult brain. A very few select areas, like the olfactory system, are the exceptions by continuing to generate new neurons throughout life. There is a very good reason for the sense of smell to retain the ability to generate new nerve cells, as will be explained later. Although the complement of neurons is largely in place at birth, their interconnections develop for a long time afterward. Similar to physical growth, full brain activation is not completed until adolescence.

Though neurons do not multiply, other cells in the brain do proliferate. Supportive cells, collectively called glial cells, are indispensable to the proper function of the brain. They nourish, sustain, maintain homeostasis, participate in signal transmission, supply nutrients and oxygen, insulate neurons, destroy pathogens and remove dead cells. As the newborn matures throughout childhood, different parts of his brain become active and fully functioning as those areas' glial cells develop and perform their functions.

The growth of glial cells is impressive. A newborn's brain weighs about 330 grm (11 oz). This is enormous considering the newborn's small body. In other mammals with a newborn of comparable size, the weight of its brain is only 30 grm (approx. 1 oz). By the infant's first birthday, the brain has more than tripled in weight to 1.1 Kg (2.4 lb). At five years old, the child's brain weighs 1.45 Kg (almost 3lb), a 420% increase from birth and is then 90% of its adult size. The majority of this increase is glial cells, which grow to ten times the number of neurons they support. The rest of the body grows too, eventually outpacing this tremendous brain growth as the human being blossoms into his neurological endowment. At birth the brain is about 9% of body weight, but as an adult it is less than 2%.

Brain function

The brain is divided into many regions denoting various functions (see figure 4.6). The three main divisions are the brain stem, the midbrain plus limbic area and the cerebrum or 'new brain', which in turn, is divided into two hemispheres.

The brain stem   The brain stem or 'old brain' so called because it is the oldest, most primitive part. It controls such basic housekeeping activities as temperature regulation, appetite, wakefulness and sleep patterns, sensory functions, cardiovascular system control, respiratory control, digestive control and pain sensitivity. All sensory and motor nerve traffic to and from the body passes through the brain stem on the way to the two cerebral hemispheres. So fundamental are these functions to living that we share them and this older brain with other animals.

The midbrain and limbic area   The midbrain controls visual and hearing reflexes and normal voluntary movement. Information flowing between brain stem and cerebrum (see below) passes through the midbrain. The limbic system

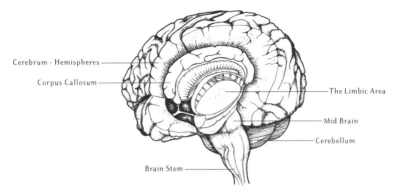

Cerebrum - Hemispheres

Corpus Callosum

The Limbic Area

Mid Brain

Cerebellum

Brain Stem

Figure 4.6 Diagrammatic representation of the brain showing location of featues mentioned in text.

involves a group of several important structures that control emotions, mood and memory functions. This area converts thoughts of the moment into those remembered for a long time. Fear, fright or flight responses, hunger, thirst, response to pain or danger, levels of pleasure, sexual satisfaction, anger and aggressive behaviour, and arousal in response to emotional circumstances are some of the aspects of our personality that are controlled by the limbic system. Parts of the limbic system combined with the olfactory nerves process information that helps associate memories to smells, regulate eating and sexual desire.

Cerebrum   We are most familiar with the cerebrum. It is the largest part and what most people think of as the brain. Intellectual conceptual ability, thinking, imagination, memory, creativity and other conscious brain functions take place within the cerebrum.

At birth there are plenty of strong connecting channels between the brain stem and midbrain called reticular formations, but not so many from midbrain to cerebrum. Of the few that do go from old brain (brain stem) through the midbrain all the way up to the cerebrum, most go to the right hemisphere and far fewer go to the left side. The developmental significance of these features will become apparent.

Of course, the entire brain is working all the time but the functions of each area have to develop fully and will do so in a precise sequential, yet overlapping manner. In the same way, a child is born with reproductive organs but they are not functional until a certain time as part of a carefully orchestrated series of events. A newborn's bones, all 330 of them, will go through a timetable of development, including some bones fusing together, until the full height and formation of the adult skeleton of 206 bones are completed.

The sequence of events generally flows from old brain to midbrain and limbic system to cerebrum with its two hemispheres. Though this is the general direction, this succession is not made up of strict delineations. As one area perfects its functioning, the next unfolding is getting ready. When new areas become active, the functions of the fully developed areas become automatic, some even working out of conscious awareness. The focus of growth on each succeeding stage necessitates withdrawing awareness or consciousness from the previous stage. For example, as old and midbrain's functional growth is completed, they perform their duties automatically without active attention, thus releasing awareness to the higher brain functions in the cerebrum where conscious, day to day thinking takes place. Without this ability of the fully developed brain functions to become automatic, progress would be delayed or cease altogether.

Summary of brain function

Putting all the pieces together, the summary of brain function looks like this. The old brain brings in raw sensory data, which then pass through the midbrain and limbic system, the centre of emotions. The pure experience gets processed, sorted and evaluated by a system of desires and preferences that creates meaningful categories. From these, the cerebrum makes creative abstractions and logical constructs. All of this is to what end? To be born means to establish existence, develop an ego, a personality, a unique self. Existence comes from the Latin word *existere* meaning to 'stand forth, appear,' and 'set apart'. That is exactly what this new life holds; the task of standing forth and establishing an identity of oneself as an ego; to set oneself apart. Looking closely at this process as it unfolds, we can see how it relates to the way we view maturation and human experience

The miniature adult

Brain growth orchestrates maturation and the innate drive to mature enhances that neurological growth. How does this affect the child's behaviour? How can understanding the child neurologically help us understand him as a whole person?

One of the most important things to understand fully is that the child is in the process of becoming a fully functioning adult, but that is many years away. It may seem self-evident, but this is a crucial point to remember. As a consequence of the child's ongoing development, his world and reality are very different from the adult world. Their needs and goals of growth are also different. It is easy to understand that a five-year-old girl has a different complement of hormones than a 25-year-old woman because their challenges and goals are different. We would no more expect a five-year-old girl to bear a child than we would expect the 25-year-old woman to have not achieved full adult height. This is patently obvious, yet this concept is often forgotten when considering the child's mental world.

Though it is known that infants feel, think and respond and that children perceive and interact with their environment, the idea that their perceptions, experiences and reactions are different than what they will later become in the years to follow has not yet been universally accepted. Typically, it is still thought that the child is simply an unformed, inexperienced or miniaturised adult. The child's view is regarded as incomplete or simply wrong, needing just the right and proper influences to be corrected and matured. It is felt that there is no particular value in the way a child thinks until he acts and experiences life correctly, meaning when his thoughts and actions resemble adults. It is quite natural to think this since the child's world eventually grows to resemble the recognisable adult one.

All too often adults see a child as a 'Mini-Me' – the same but smaller. The child is credited with using virtually the same basic thought processes and mental functioning, method of thinking, analysing, and logical processing as adults, the only difference being that they have accumulated far less raw data, experiences and facts on which to work. If there is a concept to be explained to a child, then it can be done with the same logic as an adult would understand but the vocabulary and examples just need to be simpler.

These assumptions are inaccurate. A child's world is very different from the adult one. His thoughts and behaviours, everything he senses and perceives is natural and meaningful within the context of his inner world. The child has logic, but it is the child's logic based on his own neurological functioning, perceptions, level of understanding and the needs of the stage he is in. The last influence may be the most important, because the other three are fashioned and function as a result of the needs of the stage of development.

Importance of difference

Another fundamental difference between a child's perspective and an adult's is that his world is one in which there are no boundaries or compartments between his thoughts and his experience of reality.

Adults experience the world through a complex array of abstract ideas, constructs, explanations, perceptions and ideas inherited from the past and social culture that have been unconsciously incorporated into their experience.

Adults accept these ideas as fundamentally, and often unquestioningly, true rather than being a subjective construct overlaid on the world. They convert their subjectivity into objectivity; their personal reality into universal reality.

These ideas form a boundary beyond which they rarely travel. Adults verify what they are thinking by comparing it to this pre-existing reality for confirmation and authentication. Adults ask of their thoughts, 'Does that make sense?' or 'Is this logical?'

To answer these questions, their mind is automatically flooded with a whole panoply of logical steps, experiences, knowledge, facts, formulas, images, evidence and facts against which the new experience is measured. They limit themselves by continually superimposing pre-existing ideas that colour and shape their actual experiences. This is not necessarily a bad thing. In fact, the filtering process is a very important aspect of proper brain functioning. Despite its drawbacks, without the ability to limit input by some criteria, a person would be immobilised and completely non-functional.

Adults usually judge the child's world through the same criteria of authentication that they use for their own reality. A child does not do that. Authentication is not part of his mental processing. He is able to have pure experience, appreciating it for what it is. A child's thoughts make sense and are accepted simply because he has thought them. In fact, for a child, the whole concept of making sense makes no sense. Adults and children are literally using different brains.

For the same reasons, a child's words and actions do not mean the same thing to him as they do to adults. When he says a word or exhibits some behaviour, adults automatically evaluate and interpret that within their vocabulary and experiences. In other words, adults write the dictionary for communication. Without consciously deciding, an adult automatically presupposes that the child should step into his world. He expects, even demands, that the child communicates by his rules, definitions and assumptions, correcting the child's vocabulary to slowly accommodate it to known adult terminology. It is natural to raise and educate one's child by acculturating or simply teaching him to become a healthy, active, normal person in society.

There has been a trend in the last few decades that the sooner the adaptation to the adult world happens the better off the child will be. Children are expected to enter into the adults' view of the world and functioning at an increasingly earlier age. Adult ambitions and the striving to achieve and advance in their own lives have motivated many parents to initiate education and training opportunities for their children at a young age. Whereas historically a child played at home until the age of five to six years, when they went to kindergarten if they went anywhere at all. Now it is quite common to see children start pre-school or daycare as early as one to two years old. Through their actions, adults are urging the child to 'recover' from this childhood stage as soon as possible by thinking logically and growing up to the adult world so he can get his work done.

The American educator and journalist William Lyon Phelps (1865-1943) summed up these views accurately when he said,

> 'Nature makes boys and girls lovely to look upon so they can be tolerated until they acquire some sense.'[7]

Of course, parents want the very best for their child, and encouraging the child to become mentally matured as efficiently and quickly as possible seems a good way logically to help the child. Without doubt, academic performance, skill development and achievement are highly valued and important to be a fully functioning, mature adult. The goal is not in question. It is the path and the timing to achieve that goal that needs refining.

Whatever goal parents have for their children, first they must realise that childhood is a very different stage of life than simply being an un-formed or nascent adult. Any interaction or program of learning should fully take into consideration the child's stage of development, manner of experiencing, way of thinking and processing information. The first step is to accept their vocabulary as the window to glimpse into their world. Using their particular strengths and perceptions will facilitate the child's development rather than place demands on him that he is neither physically or mentally ready to handle.

Homeopaths must do the same thing. Rather than pulling the child into our world, we should see the world from their perspective, accommodate their level of development, use their language and appreciate their way of thinking. We gain a great deal by stepping into their world with an open mind of inquiry to learn about this magical time of life.

PART TWO – ENTERING THE CHILD'S WORLD

Exploration of the child's world starts by shedding the mantle of adulthood and entering the child's world to perceive the truth of their experience. It is easier than one might imagine. For anyone who has read and enjoyed any of the Harry Potter books, you have already been there . . . and back. I suspect that the unprecedented appeal of this series of books is because they are written solely from within the child's world. Of course, there have always been children's books written from that perspective. The Harry Potter series, however, is one of the rare occasions where the child's world, in all its fantasy, creativity and imagination, is the total reality. They contain a profoundly accurate description of the world children live in. The adults and their world are the outsiders, an illogical place having no appeal whatsoever; a place the child characters want to avoid. One of the most appealing features of the books is the school and its curriculum. All the classes teach exactly what any child would love to learn. Only topics are taught that engage a child's interest and imagination and are completely divergent from the adult's logical world. Essentially, the students are being prepared to remain in the child's world, not acclimate to what appears to a child to be a very undesirable and irrelevant adult world. If only! The Harry Potter books reveal a great deal about the world in which children feel most comfortable. For adults, it is a reminder of the world they once inhabited. The Harry Potter books' phenomenal success may also be indicating that children have not spent nearly enough time there and, though still children, are longing for their own missed childhood.

Time to play

During the first seven years of a child's life, he lives in the midst of a continuous feast of new experiences and sensations, which he accumulates as the foundation of his understanding of the world (see figure 4.7).

He is constantly exploring the world and developing patterns out of what he perceives. A child is enveloped in a sensory world of touch, taste, smell, sight and sound. Children interact with the world; they touch, look, listen and taste everything around them. It is an experiential physical world; a concrete world without abstractions, concepts or logical constructs. What is – is.

Fuelled by brain and physical growth, a child incessantly explores, experiments, gathers data and receives sensory feedback from his world, especially his

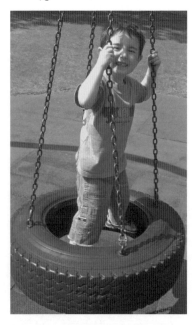

Figure 4.7 This four-year-old is busy experiencing new sensations.

parents. From all this input, he develops patterns that are meaningful to him. As they grow, children use their own special vocabulary of their known patterns to incorporate the unknown experiences into new patterns. Children make patterns; they do not question them. Very often, their patterns and vocabulary do not make any sense to us.

Children have an intense innate drive to express and expand their capacities. Their default mode is to explore, be curious and learn, expressed by what we call play. While the child plays and plays, essential changes are taking place. The 'work' of childhood is to play and fantasise; they are programmed for it. It is a misnomer to call what children do 'play' or 'fantasy'. That is the adult view. The child is simply living in his world as he perceives it, experiences it and interacts with it. He is just living. Play is life. Life is play.

Funny characters, monsters, flying people, giant beings, fairy princesses, kingdoms, talking animals, invisible friends, candy houses, plant-like people, disappearing and appearing toys, sounds, lights, music and hundreds of other parts of a child's daily reality perplex and defy our adult concept of reality and logic. What we call fantasy, a child experiences as reality.

For adults, fantasy is what does not fit into their truth of the world accumulated and formed from their years of experience and logic. From the viewpoint that the child is only an unformed and inexperienced adult-in-waiting, the childhood fantasy world of play seems unimportant or a waste of time. The parental urge is to structure the child's play, provide educational toys, TV programmes and generally make good 'use' of this time. Often the child's unbending tendency to play confronts the adult idea of what is appropriate to do, what the 'real' learning of life is. Only in the adult world is there a differentiation between play and work, where play is purposeless fun and work is productive but usually unpleasant. The child experiences no such division. He just lives, learns, explores and enjoys. (Maybe adults should be learning from him!)

From the view that Nature plans for success, this playful time of life has its own very special purpose. Perpetual playing results in proper brain growth and functioning. After the age of seven, the innate urges and desires for experience automatically change the child's play to encompass another phase of learning – logical organisation of the world. What happens next will depend on how extensive and strong is the framework laid down in these earlier years of play. It is hoped that it has been formed thoroughly since it must hold up the entire edifice of the person's adult world for the rest of his life.

Homeopaths should have some measure of empathy for the child's imaginative world being overshadowed by the dictate of adult logic. After all, the behemoth of modern medicine represented by allopaths insists that homeopaths live in a fantasy world because their ideas are not logical and make no sense according to science and physics. Of course, homeopaths think that allopaths live in a barren, closed one-dimensional world because they think the body and mind are not connected and that health has nothing to do with a person's emotional or spiritual life. Setting our discord aside, the point is that we do have logic but it is a different kind of logic than the allopaths use. We perceive the world differently than they do and our ideas are based on that perspective. It has its place and function. Similarly, children have a different kind of logic than adults, proper in its own right and its own place.

The best thing to do for a child is to rely on his innate drive for expansion and growth to move him forward to maximum mental health and development. Adults do not feel the urge to instruct the child's bone cells how to deposit calcium, or tell the newborn's heart when it is time to close the *ductus arteriosus* or tell the fingers how to grasp. There is confidence that physical growth will proceed automatically according to plan. As long as the child gets good food and is in a safe, loving environment, Nature will take care of the rest.

Yet, with the child's mental development there is not that same confidence that everything will proceed correctly for the child's welfare without constant intervention and supervision. The fact remains that the drive for mental growth and development is just as precise, vigorous and undaunted as it is for physical growth. As with physical growth, all that is needed for optimum mental development is to provide the nutrients and a healthy, loving, stimulating and supportive environment. Let the child function and the structure of learning will take care of itself. Awareness, consciousness or intelligence is not given to the child. Innate qualities and capacities flourish when the needed conditions are established or supported. It is telling that the fastest rate of learning; the most profound, extensive, fruitful and fundamental learning, of immense complexity and significance takes place in the first three years of life, without formal instruction and when the child is not aware that what is happening is learning.

The child will thrive, until and unless his natural drives are thwarted and destroyed. So strong is that inner drive of curiosity and exploration that it takes a lot of effort to incapacitate or obliterate it. A child who is not interested in learning is an anomaly. Curiosity and the imaginative facility are so natural to childhood that its absence is startling to behold.

I recall one such instance. I was walking on the grounds of a local hotel famous for its beautiful series of ponds, walkways, bridges, streams and the number of resident swans. I was standing on one of the wooden bridges over a pool, watching the swans leisurely floating with their serene majesty. Two children about seven and eight years old joined me to observe the swans. They pointed and watched with obvious interest and we began talking about the swans. At one point I asked them what they imagined it would be like to be a swan. Bewildered, the children stared at me. They appeared to have no idea what I was talking about. I repeated the question but they still seemed confused. Finally the older of the two said, 'But we aren't swans.' They just could not release logic enough to allow their imagination to take wing. I found it almost impossible to imagine a child who cannot imagine. Logic sat far too comfortably on their slender shoulders. Even at their young age, already their innate ability to experience their child's world was stifled to the extent of being incapable to become a swan. Where was their playfulness, their ability to invent, dream and envision? I wondered what kind of education they must have had that could so successfully extinguish a child's normal faculty of imagination. What could have happened?

Moving and thinking

The answer to that question lies in understanding the way young children learn best. The faculty to learn is not separate from growing, breathing, moving, smiling or living. It does not take place in a special place called school; everything a child experiences teaches something. In fact, learning does not take place only in the brain: the child thinks with his whole body. His action is his thinking and his thinking makes his actions. Learning is kinaesthetic and must include actual participation in a physical activity involving active body movement. Living as he does in a sensory world, his senses must be used to learn. This means interacting with the world around him by picking things up, tasting them, examining them, throwing them, shaking them, touching them and taking things apart. His is a hands-on world. By interacting in an experiential way, he tries, gets feedback, restructures, tries again and learns.

Learning must have interaction with things; it does not occur with passivity. A child's mind is not designed to learn that way. Being passive breaks the loop of exploration, feedback and re-exploration. Listening or watching a demonstration or the television does not utilise the full sensory, movement experience and interaction necessary for the best learning. Children often hate school because they are forced to learn but deprived of the ability because they are not allowed to move. Children move constantly because they are learning constantly. Children cannot sit still because learning takes place with physical muscular activity.

René Descartes' (1596–1650) famous dictum, *Je pense donc je suis*[8] translated as *'I think, therefore I am'* could be modified for children to, 'I move therefore I think.'

This must be kept in mind before rushing to use the following rubric:

- MIND; Restlessness, in children

Active play is the movement needed to develop to stimulate the building of neuron circuits and develop the child's brain. It is essential to develop thinking capacities, which is the foundation of later learning. The child's drive to explore precedes and helps develop his abilities. Increasing abilities then develop his brain. The more the child learns, the more he can learn. Stimulation increases the brain's capacity for more stimulation. Providing a child with an interesting and stimulating environment enhances the innate flexibility of the brain and its capacities and is essential to proper growth and development.

Too much of a good thing

A note of caution is that there can be too much of a good thing. Many times adults think they are enabling and propelling a child forward by providing them with an enhanced environment of stimulation. The majority of the time this is correct, however, this is not always the case. The stimulation must be of the right type at the right time in the right amount – when the brain is ready to process it. It is vital to interact with the child at his level of cognitive development. Learning can be inhibited by blocking the child's interaction with the new and unknown and equally by providing experiences that are inappropriate for age and therefore cannot be assimilated. If the environment created for the child is designed for the adults' goals, then the child does not have the opportunity to structure it at his pace. Stimulation at the wrong time or of the wrong kind leads to anxiety and withdrawal. Some educational toys promote responses the child's mind is not matured enough to provide. Often logical thinking is needed to interact with the toys, when the child's best facilities are imagination and play.

It is obvious that a six-year-old is not mentally ready for the challenge of high school, or a 10-year-old would not function well in college any more than either could lift 100 kg (220 lb) Their mental capacities are not yet equipped for those levels. It is equally true in more subtle ways; a six-year-old is not best suited for most academic pursuits or the development of logical reasoning. He might appear to perform well enough because he can do it to a certain extent. However, at this stage his brain development is not fully ready for those lessons. Further-more, the precise unfolding of the developmental timetable is being altered. He is jumping ahead, missing out on the full flowering of other important stages of his neurological and mental maturation. His efforts are best suited to imagina-tive play, socialising and following his natural curiosity. He is learning a great deal, but from a framework that is different than the logical constraints of formal academics.

Innate timetable

Many parents have the concern that a child allowed to remain in the world of make-believe will never move out of it to the world of logic and adult conceptual and analytical thinking. That is not the case. The child himself moves through the learning stages at his own pace and will enact his desire to develop adult style thinking as naturally and seamlessly as learning to walk or learning to run. For example, part of childhood is the story of Santa Claus bringing presents at Christmas time or the Tooth Fairy redeeming a fallen tooth for a coin during the night. These are good examples of times when adults do step into a child's reality. For a child, Santa Claus is quite real. It does not at all enter a child's mind to question his existence just because there are dozens of different Santa Clauses around town, or that he has to give gifts to all children worldwide during one night.

Both of these familiar residents of the child's universe begin to fade away around the age of seven to eight as the child shifts more and more to the adult world through his development of logical thinking. As the child exercises more analytical abilities, the 'logic' about Santa being many different adults dressing up intrudes and finally overtakes his child's world experience of Santa as a magical being. Most children come to work this out for themselves as their mental equipment advances to the point of making these conclusions. It is interesting that the first deciduous tooth comes out at about age six, well within the age for the Tooth Fairy to have existence but before the time when imagination begins to give way to logic and analysis. During the ensuing years, more teeth continue to fall. By the age of 12, not only have all the deciduous teeth fallen out because the child has outgrown them, but he has also outgrown the Tooth Fairy. Adult logic and analytic processing have taken over as the primary mental function.

Child's logic and the adult logic are very different ways of processing information and sensory experiences. In many ways, a child's way of learning is the same as a tenured university professor doing basic research. Both explore and investigate for the sheer joy of learning and discovery and go wherever their curiosity takes them. The child is rapidly gathering experiences, data, information and a myriad of seemingly unrelated thoughts and ideas, all of which expand his world and strengthen his mind. A child does not evaluate his actions by the yardstick of utility, usefulness, purposefulness or 'making the research pay'. Childhood is not a time for survival concerns or utility. Those demands have their proper time and place, belonging to a later stage fully integrated into the adult world. Pursuing those concerns at the wrong time creates stress, fear and inhibition. Without doubt, all the information gathered with such random abandon will have a useful part to play in later development, just as basic research provides the fundamental building blocks of knowledge that is later used for specific purposes.

Learning to walk provides a good example of how seemingly unrelated antecedent actions contribute to the later benefits. It is easy to understand logically how standing and stepping are necessary contributors to obtaining the skill of walking, as is how the infant's action of rolling over from back to front and front to back has its place in the developmental continuum towards walking. What is not so obviously connected to walking is the child waving his arms around, suckling or grasping at our outstretched hand. These actions too are laying the groundwork for neurological, visual and muscular exercise and coordination essential for walking.

The childhood years are a time for the child to explore his world of play and imagination, establishing a firm foundation before expanding his possibilities into the world of logical thinking. The precursor to proficient logical thinking is not a simpler form of logic: it is fantasy and imagination. The connection may be hard to make logically, nonetheless, the non-logical playful, imaginative stage of childhood is the foundation from which logical adults arise. I say expand rather than replace, because the ability to imagine, perceive the non-logical and comprehend the irrational are important brain functions that ought not to be lost. Though still present in adults, they are usually completely tyrannised by logic and rational constructs. A human being's full potential includes being comfortable and proficient in both worlds rather than submerging one to the complete favour of the other.

The depth of time vision

There are some additional physical and mental changes in childhood that are relevant to the homeopathic treatment of children. Children live in a world of 'here and now and me'. A child knows the place he is in is 'here', the time is 'now' and everything in that 'here and now' relates to him. As the child grows, his 'here and now and me' expands to include other places, other times and other people. The 'now' aspect of the child's experience is his sense of time. The perception of time as it relates to children and maturation is an important concept to understand, with far reaching ramifications in development, education, parenting and homeopathic treatment. How much time can a child understand? How far into the future can a child recognise and consider? How far or 'deep' his time perception goes changes with growth and is a good indicator of development.

Time is the grid on which people rest, so naturally it is assumed that all people see it the same way. Adults and children, however, experience time in significantly different ways. Long before Einstein mathematically demonstrated the inconsistency of time with his Theory of Relativity, many people had experienced the elasticity of time. Time is not an inviolate uniform measure; it is how life is experienced. How does time function throughout childhood?

Intrauterine life is a timeless world. The foetus has continual food and nutrients, constant temperature and stability. There is no conscious awareness of yesterday or tomorrow, this minute or that minute. There is nothing to mark one moment from the next. Even the mother's heartbeat is less a metronome than it is part of the stable, comforting endlessness. There is just peaceful, time-less existence.

Time begins at the moment of birth. The adult sense of time is expressed when the day and precise moment of a child's birth is noted. The newborn's experience is very different; he has to breathe and breathe now. In the immedi-acy of that split second of his new life, the newborn has to breathe on his own and keep breathing every few seconds. Breathing is one of the many urgent changes that occur at birth. His awareness of time is purely physiological. His is a world of immediacy and urgency where even seconds matter. Physical mech-anisms for any delay or future considerations are not available yet. The newborn cannot regulate his own body temperature so he needs constant external temperature regulation. His body has very little ability to store food, so he must eat very frequently or he will run out of nutrients and fluids. He needs to be constantly with his mother so he can receive breast milk many times throughout the day, even several times an hour. The newborn is designed to have these frequent small meals necessitating closeness to his mother because they coincide with other important developmental features such as skin stimulation, constant exposure to his mother's heartbeat and face. All aspects of newborn life revolve around moment to moment living. His time frame is very short indeed.

As the physical changes in the newborn occur to allow longer time between meals and greater amounts of waking time, his time reference is also extending. Soon the infant will have the depth of time vision extending to hours. He ex-periences the world as binary, 'either-or'; hot or cold, hungry or satiety; comfort-able or uncomfortable. When one of his needs requires attending, it still must be done with some promptness but he can function from hour to hour with confi-dence.

During the first year, the infant's short time reference means 'out of sight, out of mind'. He has no object permanency because his time frame is not long enough. The child can be easily distracted because the time reference is so short. At another age, this might be called attention deficit, but at this age it is expected.

At about 12 months a child develops the sense of object permanency. Things in the world, including the mother, can be assumed to be there from one moment to the next, one day to the next. This is such a momentous milestone with far reaching significance for the child's development, that it will be discussed in more detail later. It is mentioned here because the ability to perceive the permanency of an object, in addition to an indicator of neurological development, is a sign of the increasing length of time reference. Things can exist in time because there is a perception of time. With permanence the child does not have to re-establish a safe place every day. Now his intelligence and curiosity can investigate other things from this safe place.

Two and three-year-olds operate with a one-day time reference. What happens today is all that matters. The daily routine is understood and expected. The still short depth of time perception means children of this age feel more comfortable and secure with stable, consistent and unvaried environments on a day-to-day basis. Object permanency is now part of the child's familiar world, so small variations can be met with security. When a mother states that her child does not like change, she might equally say her child's depth of time vision is very short.

At ages three to four the child can perceive a future of several days. Concepts of yesterday, tomorrow and the day after have meaning in his life. By age 6, he can understand the idea of a week. At this age many children are in school 5 days a week. The concept of a week being Monday to Friday in school with a weekend tagged on at the end is understandable and experienced. Anything too far beyond a week is all the same; some amorphous nebulous place a long way away and a long time from now.

It is helpful to understand a child's time frame of reference. This is not a matter of education; it is a matter of brain development and function. Experiencing time differently happens automatically as the child's physical and mental processes develop. To communicate more effectively with a child, step into the child's world and use his time reference.

For a four or five-year-old, having a 'time out' or being required to wait for more than 10 minutes, is like a whole day for an adult. Rewarding a six-year-old's behaviour with the promise of a present next week is incomprehensible. A reward later in the same day would work.

Children at ages seven to nine start understanding and experiencing periods of a year; that there are annual events like Christmas and birthdays and summer time. Though they understand this conceptually because their logic is developing at this time, they do not yet fully experience this length of time. For a child of this age, a delay of a year would not fit in their time reference. Saving money for college is not likely to meet with enthusiasm, but saving money for a weekend treat or a special event in several weeks' or months' time would have meaning.

After age nine, the perception of time continues to lengthen. Pre-teens operate on an annual time frame. Children of this age are often asked, 'What school class or grade are you in?' and 'When is your birthday?' both references to yearly events. This does not mean that nine-year-olds do not understand about years, decades or centuries. They can intellectually understand a longer time than they experience in their life. The ability to work today for something tomorrow, delayed gratification, is seen as a good sign of maturity. It is more accurately called the increasing depth of time vision. It requires the ability to think in terms of months, years or decades to be able to value the concept of delaying a reward to a later time. In other words, future years have to exist before the person can imagine something happening then.

Determining the depth of time perception for any patient is helpful to understand from which stage of development he may be operating his life. Is he a precocious 10-year-old already thinking about his future profession and his college years, or is he a 40-year-old living pay cheque to pay cheque and unable to save any money? Often after successful homeopathic treatment, the patient lives more in his age-appropriate time frame.

There are several rubrics with reference to time perception:

- MIND; Time, passes too slowly
- MIND; Time, loss of the conception of
- MIND; Time, passes too quickly
- MIND; Mistakes in time

Though not as detailed as is needed to be useful, they can help in some adult cases. Referring to the first two rubrics listed, 14% of the remedies are from the second and third row of the periodic table, which contain remedies representing childhood stages of life.

The process of lengthening time perception does not end after childhood; it continues throughout life. It is worth mentioning that teens, young adults, adults, mid-life adults and the elderly all have different depths of time vision. Young adults think in terms of several years and adults usually experience their life in three to five year segments. Mid-life adults start celebrating only their decade birthdays: 40, the 'big four-oh' and 50, the 'big five-oh'. The decades seem to pass with increasing speed and fluidity; ten years pass as quickly as one used to. Investment for the future and saving for retirement begins to be more of a concern as the depth of time vision spans decades. For the later years after 60, the time reference is generational and with grandchildren being part of life. What legacy will be left behind to the next generation? Maybe those who can see so far down the tunnel of time that they have generational concerns on their minds enjoy the company of young children because it is refreshing to be reminded of a time when the whole world could be experienced in a single day.

Newborn – changing worlds
Existence consciousness

As described, the neural tissue starts forming just weeks after conception. Over the ensuing months, these original rudimentary cells quickly proliferate and organise. At about four to six months, the nervous system is mature enough to control some body functions. This marks the point of accelerated brain growth and development, revealing evidence of hearing and responsive movements. The intrauterine world is a stable environment muffled in darkness and quiet. All potential sensory input from our world is muted, yet not totally eliminated. Encased in a protective waxy insulation while floating in the quiet, dark, warm watery world, the growing foetus has very little sensory stimulation. He only experiences the constant subdued stimulation of the mother's heartbeat, voice, breathing, internal organ movements and the rocking of her many movements. Only the senses needed in such a protected place are activated.

Birth is a series of sequential steps that results in the foetus leaving intrauterine existence to enter life as an infant. The process starts with the first stirrings in the foetus as his stable, comfortable intrauterine existence becomes limiting. From his established safe place, he experiences the urging to expand into unknown territory.

The change to an entirely different environment at birth establishes the immediate need to activate other sensory and neurological functions. The brain is waiting expectantly for the appropriate signals to start the next cascade of development. Full sensory activation cannot start before there is sensory stimulation. It is as if there is a switch that needs to be turned on but that only life outside of the uterus can do. Activation of the senses and their neurological connections must be carried out for the newborn. He cannot provide himself with sensory stimulation. He requires interaction.

The very first stimulus and neurological change to the newborn is to breathe and that happens in a very short time frame. So critical is this transition, that Nature provides dual oxygen for the first minutes of life. After birth, oxygen is still being delivered through the umbilical cord but now a new source is added, the newborn's lungs, thereby giving time for the crucial neurological, sensory and respiratory functions to work properly. Another protection against an interruption in oxygen supply is the special resistance a newborn's brain cells have to fluctuating oxygen levels, far more resilient that at any other time of life. Even with these protective mechanisms, many newborns suffer subtle forms of hypoxemia in this transition; too subtle for medical science's testing but enough to affect the oxygen-sensitive brain cells.

Activation of the newborn's full array of sensory apparatus is the next import-ant stage of development. Smell, touch, sight, hearing, taste in addition to balance, proprioception, neuromuscular coordination and other functions must be activated and developed. Touch is a critical ingredient (see figure 4.8). The skin is highly sensitive with its billions of nerve endings. Everything from simple touch to gentle massaging, holding, caressing, touching and skin contact is required to stimulate the brain to develop all its activities. The brain is designed to depend on extensive skin stimulation for its initial activation and proper development. This point cannot be emphasised enough.

Figure 4.8 shows a mother holding her newborn son with an elder daughter. It was taken in an allopathic maternity hospital – an environment in which most mothers routinely find themselves. This does not necessarily preclude the use of homeopathy – a box of remedies may be seen on the bedside cabinet. The half-smile on the sibling's face may reflect some apprehension about a new 'competi-tor' for her parents' affection

Many hormones are involved in pregnancy, birth and lactation in both mother and child, which interact in complex ways. A few are distinctly related to the newborn's development. Though a natural process, birth is stressful and potentially traumatic for the infant. Therefore, it is not surprising that the newborn releases the stress hormones adrenaline and cortisone to assure the physiological support needed during this time. With proper skin stimulation through contact with the mother, the comfort of hearing her heartbeat, her warmth, breast-feeding and maternal production of oxytocin, all signal that the stressful journey has ended in a very safe place allowing the stress hormones to drop back to normal levels. With a healthy, normal birth, the infant will smile within the first hour of his new life.

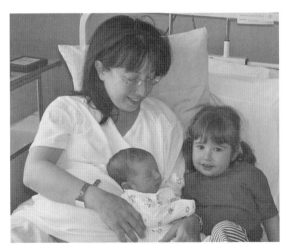

Figure 4.8 Touch is a critical ingredient for the newborn.

If the expected calming influences of reassurance, safety and protection are not forthcoming at this time, then the infant continues to experience enough stress to maintain high levels of cortisone. Cortisone is designed to enact the body and mind functions necessary to cope with and get out of stress or crisis. Such physiological and mental changes are not intended for normal daily life. Cortisone acts like an overdraft facility on a bank account which is intended to help out in an emergency but not to pay the normal expenses. Long time administration cortisone is very harsh and debilitating. It stops growth and learning because it keeps the body and mind in a state of alarm, tension and fear.

Many aspects of our western medical birthing practices perpetuate the presence of high levels of cortisone in the newborn, with undesirable consequences. The infant's first hours and days remain tense and stressful. The beautiful newborn smile is missing; after all there is nothing to smile about. He cannot process the incoming sensory signals to full advantage, and he will not manage to initiate the expected array of neurological functions. It is possible that prolonged high adrenaline and cortisone in the time immediately after birth may be establishing the 'set point' for the child's life, thereby requiring a lifetime of stress and tension to maintain the levels that were imprinted as a newborn.

Humans are social beings. A happy, productive life, even our very survival, depends on other people. Essential socialisation starts right at birth. Bonding with people starts from the first moments of life. The newborn's brain is already programmed to recognise and respond to a human face. Many hours of his early life are spent staring at one particular face – his mother's. The infant's position for nursing is perfect to gaze at her. This position has other developmental functions. In addition to providing nourishment, the infant is closest to the mother's heartbeat. Experienced since the moment of conception, this ultimately familiar sound now helps his acclimation to a new world of unfamiliar sensory experiences. The jaw movement of suckling in this position helps activate the ear, balance and the ability to orient sounds in space.

Even the qualities of human milk support the expected stages of neurological and physical development. Human milk is far more dilute than that of other mammals, necessitating the infant to nurse frequently for his required nutrients. This dovetails perfectly with the infant's developmental needs of close maternal contact, frequent skin stimulation and massage, face recognition and other sensory input.

Our understanding of the newborn during its first months of life has undergone tremendous change. Until very recently, the newborn was regarded as an undifferentiated organism lacking perception, sensation, intelligence, conscious experience of the world or any psychological functions. The bundle of joy was just a bundle. For several months the bundle simply alternated between a sleeping vegetative state and a waking vegetative state. Finally, after a few months, the first faint signs of conscious awareness began to emerge. From this perspective, it is easy to understand why it was presumed that human infants were born 3 months before they were ready for the world. Their 'obvious' lack of any intelligence or consciousness was because they should have been completing their mental development *in utero*, which unfortunately was not possible. The increase in human intelligence necessitated such a large head that the infant had to be born prematurely in order to be born at all. Nature clearly had made a mistake. She simply forgot to change the human female's pelvis bone architecture to allow for the infant's enlarging head. I am always surprised when a theory depends on the assumption that Nature got it wrong. As if it were really possible that the most critical part of any species existence, successful reproduction, was reduced to a matter of carelessly overlooking a necessary line item on some cosmic to-do list.

The publication of Frederick LeBoyer's groundbreaking book entitled *Birth without Violence*, in 1974[9] was a turning point for the dawning awareness about the reality of an infant's prenatal life, its birth and newborn life. Most people now realise that the newborn is a highly intelligent, responsive, experience gathering and integrated human being. With a brain five times larger in ratio to its body size in comparison to adults, there is obviously a lot of mental activity possible and necessary. We have come that far in acknowledging that the infant, even before birth, is fully alive, sentient, and responsive.

First year – sensory world
Separation consciousness

The first year of life has many changes, some of which have been mentioned. During the entire year, the infant establishes a sensory connection to both environment and basic bodily functions. This is the province of the old brain – incorporating basic brain functions and a physical sensory system. All these functions are the basic workings of the mind and body and must be developed and fully functional before the next step can be made. Think of this stage as a computer getting its operating system installed. The operating system is what makes the whole computer work, booting up the computer and keeping it running smoothly, performing its functions in the background no matter what other actions the computer is performing. It has specific essential functions of its own, but mainly it allows all other programs to work.

The infant is helpless and completely dependent its first year, to the extent that all sensory experiences are provided for him, usually by the mother. Though he is not yet able to initiate his own explorations, he stills needs to experience and learn to function on this earthly realm. As the infant grows he becomes more stabilised and familiar in his new environment. His brain stem has filled in the

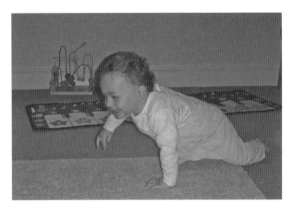

Figure 4.9 The ability to crawl gives the child sensory input beyond his immediate available world.

basic information about the world, so he begins to want to venture to explore on his own, initiate his own search for sensory input and seek new and interesting things to encounter. The innate urge propels the child onward outside his existing world of immediately available sensory experience, manifesting by the ability to crawl (see figure 4.9).

Years one to four – self assertion
Identity consciousness

The infant starts to move around in his environment, all controlled by brain stem activity. After one year these functions become automatic, creating a level of autonomy and functional independence. The next phase is unfolding as his midbrain and limbic system take centre stage. These brain structures control functions of the will and emotional drives, likes and dislikes, judgement of sensory experiences, mood and preferences, pleasure and happiness. It is the task of the midbrain and limbic system to put an emotional overlay to pure sensory data supplied by the brain stem; to take sensations and make meaning-ful relationships, categories and patterns. Judgement and an evaluative process unfold. Seeing becomes perception. General becomes specific.

All sensory data comes through the brainstem except the sense of smell. Instead of being located in the old brain along with other senses, smell functions with the midbrain and limbic system. This neurological home ground demon-strates the connection between smell and other limbic system functions such as bonding, pleasure and emotions. Smell affects sexuality through pheromones. From an embryological connection, smell is related to the immune system – the basic ability to tell self from not self. Recall that the olfactory neurons retain their ability to multiply. The immune system needs the ability to be mutable and expandable as the immune needs change, which may account for the flexibility preserved by olfactory neurons. With the sense of smell linked to so many important emotional functions, it is understandable why it is interconnected with the limbic structures.

The shift of consciousness to the midbrain and limbic areas is coincident with the lengthening of time perception. Starting at one year of age, the child's entire world changes with the momentous development of object consistency. Though usually occurring without any fanfare, it is as big of a milestone as the more celebrated teething, walking or puberty. Object consistency facilitates the child's ability to experience his environment as stable and familiar. From that solid ground, he can venture out to experiment with his world by being emotional, wilful and self-assertive. Language now develops as another way of putting sensory experiences into categories. The child stands, walks, names things, wants things and is exerting a will of his own.

With sensory data coming in at all moments, the midbrain and limbic system are very busy. Not only is it necessary to categorise everything into useful and meaningful order, but also values and preferences are being developed so that the brain can judge and choose what is valuable information. One of the most important functions of categorising is to discard information. Conscious awareness is forged out of an infinite number of possibilities for attention. There is always far more sensory input than we can manage, irrespective of our stage of development. In order to cope with the massive amount of data and organise it to be useful, we judge and choose some options and not others. Out of necessity some possibilities must be cut off. We must decide. From the Latin *decidere*, decide, it literally means 'to cut off'.

Life would be confusing and simply immobilising without this function. Most people have had a small taste of this process in trying to cope with the information age. How could anyone hope to be able to manage muddling through the vast amount of currently available information? How could all newspapers, journals and books be read, all available video programs be seen, all upcoming research and available knowledge that is expanding hourly be reviewed; let alone analysed and synthesised to be useful? Obviously it cannot. A strategy of information sorting and filtering must be used to permit a person to concentrate only on the most valuable. Like a computer email program, a spam filter is needed. Remember the time, not too long ago, when email in-boxes were inundated with hundreds or thousands of unwanted messages? Despite their complete uselessness, it still took time to manually filter through them. Now there are computer functions that automatically do that, called spam filters. The human brain does the same thing for basically the same reason. The miracle of the brain is that it can make filters that eliminate data, yet at the same time it stays flexible and inclusive.

Adults cannot be faulted for having preconceived ideas and ignoring the new and innovative. No one would ever have become an adult if there had not been some kind of filtering system. The price paid for it is that the majority of the wide range of open possibilities is cut out. Sometimes our filtering works too well and the new, unfamiliar and challenging is lost.

Infants and young children do not do this, at least not yet. They can allow more in because the brain areas that limit sensory input are not fully functioning yet. The ability to organise sensory data, and to selectively cut out most of it is based on an emotional overlay, on judgement and preferences. Placing the rest into meaningful categories is the task of the parts of the brain that are now developing. The child is learning to choose one sensory experience in preference to another. He still interacts with the myriad of possibilities as in his first year. Now, however, he exerts his will, emotions and preferences by deciding in favour of some experiences over others.

Aristotle observed,

'The life of children is wholly governed by their desires.'

That is as it should be. Through his physical body, the child experiences the sensory world; his reactions are based on emotions, values, choices and preferences. His investigations require that he decide preferences; yes or no; this or that; like or dislike; good or bad. He is ascribing value and that means having a sense of ego, an identity. It is the 'I' that decides, prefers and chooses. The power of decision is the power of identity. The ability to decide is the ability to be independent, to be oneself. The emergence of a personal identity, exercising personal choice and experiencing personal power are essential aspects to become a whole, healthy, vital person. Knowledge of the physical world through interaction with it gets integrated through conscious judgement. The result is self-awareness and self-consciousness and a crucial ability to form an identity.

The very beginning of a sense of individuality or identity starts when choice is introduced to differentiate experiences from the sameness of the vast sensory input. When the child makes a single choice, he has created and individualised his universe. His universe is no longer the same as anyone else's. The midbrain and limbic system facilitate this expression of individual identity.

Though the child is learning to evaluate and choose, he is not fully autonomous. Parental influences of support, displeasure, encouragement and role modelling play key roles in his decisions. Generally his choices will favor those experiences that have the widest array of full sensory information as well as parental support.

Many parents get frustrated when their three-year-old learns to say 'no'. Once learned, every comment, suggestion or request seems to be met with their now favourite word, 'NO!' Recall that words do not mean the same thing to children as they do to adults. 'No' in the adult world means just that, 'no'. For the child, saying 'no' is the exercising of new brain functions - those of choice and identity. Every 'no' holds the claim of the emerging identity to its rightful place as an individual. Identity is so important to being a healthy person that its development starts at a very early age. The 'terrible twos' are really the limbic system overlaying emotions to the child's experiences by asserting his will and establishing his identity.

It has taken the three years from ages one to four for the midbrain and limbic system to activate and coordinate its functions. At the end of this phase, about 80% of knowledge of the physical world's structure, language and ego awareness is complete. Once this stage is achieved the child is ready to move to the next phase – activation and incorporation of the cerebrum while simultaneously the midbrain and limbic structure functions will become automatic, below conscious awareness.

Age four – bridging the mind
Family consciousness

Now that the child has established his identity and the majority of his verbal skills he can do more for himself. The child at this age becomes more interested in the immediate surroundings outside of himself – his family. He no longer is living solely in a world of his own making; those other very familiar people are involved. Though he is growing to include others, his world is still circumscribed within the bounds of family. With an identity, he can form bonds, interact with others and participate in ongoing relationships. He is less dependent and passive now, being able to exert his desires and personality in the interactions. The stability and safety of the family affords him this area of growth and maturation.

A very important phase of brain growth is also occurring. The most advanced part of the brain, the cerebrum, has two separate hemispheres, connected by a neural bridge called the corpus callosum (see figure 4.6). All messages from one side to the other must pass through this bridge. For the first year of life, it is small and mostly dormant, thereby limiting communication between the sides. There is little need for much communication between the hemispheres because both sides undergo parallel development. Each gets all the same information about basic whole body functions imported from the brainstem through the midbrain, which serves as the only functional connection between the two sides. Until this stage is mostly completed, learning differs from what it will be later when communication between the sides is possible.

At the end of the first year of life, there is a shift of activity to the midbrain and limbic system. This necessitates contact between the two sides; consequently, the corpus callosum begins to grow and become active. It is slow in developing and does not fully complete its growth until about three or four years of age. This is of major significance – the two sides of the new brain can begin to communicate directly without involving the midbrain.

As the child enters this phase of development, there already is a multitude of connections from brainstem to right hemisphere but far less to the left side. The right side gets all the information straight from the brainstem through the midbrain. The result is that the right-brain function is developed first. It processes and stores information as imagery, fantasy, whole pictures, body motions and creative play – a pre-logic way of experiencing life.

The left hemisphere's main functions of logic, analysis and abstract thinking are not needed in the child's early years, therefore it makes sense that there are fewer neural pathways directly to and from the brainstem and midbrain. In this stage, information traffic from those areas to the left brain must pass first through the unifying processing of the right brain. This cannot begin to happen until there is a pathway between the hemispheres, which becomes active after the first birthday. However, it is not until the corpus callosum is fully formed and functional, at about age four that this pathway can contribute significantly to the child's development. Once that happens logic, conceptual and abstract thought can be used to further process incoming data. A very subtle and elegant way of orchestrating neurological development, it means that the logical processing happens only after the right brain has been utilised and developed for some years. It is usually thought that our cultures do not allow enough right brain functions to be developed. The right brain develops faster than the left by several years and is therefore more fully developed sooner. Far from not allowing right brain development, it is more accurate to say that in a person's later years its developed functions are overshadowed by too much left brained, logical thought.

Once the two hemispheres are able to communicate easily with each other they can specialise into different functions. Without such means of communication between the two sides, a division of mental labour could not exist. Each side would have to continue to perform all functions, as they do in the first year of life. We might joke about chaotic office staff by saying that 'The right hand does not know what the left one is doing,' but that is exactly what would happen to a person if there were no corpus callosum. If all functions were carried out in both hemispheres, the size of the brain and its energy consumption would be much larger, which is neither efficient nor practical. Nature is not that wasteful. Fortunately we do have the communication bridge and as a result, we have developed a much more versatile and functional brain through specialisation.

The left side of the brain specialises in logic, language and digital sequential concepts. The right specialises in abstract, creative, analogue, whole-picture functions. The left side reads sequentially; the right side takes in the entire picture at once. Roughly speaking, the left is for logic and the right side is for patterns. For example, the left brain is used to tell the time from a digital watch; the right brain is used to tell the time from a watch with a dial and two hands. Digital and analog; numbers and forms; logic and creativity; sequential and whole; both are necessary, each side being a compliment to the other.

When someone has retained or re-enlivened this right brain imaginative quality, we regard them as someone with a special creative talent like an artist, fiction writer or craftsman. However, the fully realised person is conversant with all aspects of themselves and uses both sides of the brain. This development begins in childhood.

Age four to seven
Creativity consciousness

After the age of four, learning is different to previous stages because different equipment is becoming operational. Mainly, the cerebrum with its two hemi-spheres and the connection between, the corpus callosum, are added in a very robust and exciting way. Until now, his right brain development has been more than left, but the upcoming phase serves to develop left brain activity. The child is still exploring the world around him with vigour and unceasing curiosity but his playground has expanded and he can use, practice and play with his 'new toy' – his integrated, imaginative and creative mind.

The child's ego and intellect emerge and solidify at this stage of development. These years are a time of 'pre-reasoning' concrete thinking directly related to his 'here and now and me' physical and sensory experience. He lives in a subjective world. All that is important is the 'what is it' and what he feels about it. The 'why is it' or logical thinking will come later.

Coming on the heels of his creative fantasy world based on concrete sensory experiences, this phase moves a step further to include intuitive creative thinking and abstract imagery and thought. All thought is imagery: all reality is imagery. The language skills already mastered serve his imagination by using words to link his experience to the imagery in his mind. Now is a time for stories, metaphor, analogies, symbols such as Santa Claus, kings and princesses, magic powers and super heroes and other strong icons created out of an imaginary world.

The Spanish philosopher and poet George Santayana (1863–1952) observed,

> 'Children are natural mythologists: they beg to be told tales, and love not only to invent but to enact falsehoods.'[10]

The child needs to imagine and create for himself, to develop the ability to make his own imagery. To create for oneself is an aspect of identity development. In earlier years, the child's identity was founded on the ability to make his choice out of what already existed. Now his identity is further developed by creating what did not exist before.

Maybe Descartes' dictum mentioned above needs another variation, 'I create, therefore I am.'

Through this process the child is building up a capacity for creating through his imagination. His images are now less concrete and more fluid and powerful, preparing the way for the left-brain's prowess of abstract thought.

Asking 'why' at age five means something different than at age 15. The best approach is to answer according to the brain function at that age. For example, about the age of five, children often ask about death. Many parents get concerned about what seems to be a sad and morbid preoccupation in their child. Another way to see this is as a part of developing an identity. Identity means one exists as a unique individual. Along with the experience of existing comes the opposite, the idea of not existing or the concept of death. For the child of five, the concept of death is about identity, exerting choice, existing as an individual and saying 'I am here'.

This imaginative playful time of life is critically important as a foundation for further growth. At the end of this phase, the child prepares for a shift from his own self-made playground of imagination to the social world of other people and the logical constructs required to interact with them. His subjective is about to become objective.

Age seven to eleven – abstract thinking
Social consciousness

The age of seven marks a time of great brain growth resulting in a major functional shift in the child's mental development to more left brain activity, thereby bringing new skills, perspectives and dramatically increased mental capacities. The right hemisphere's functions of non-logical imagery and creativity are now automatic. They are so essential to proper left brain logical thinking that they have been perfected first.

Up to this time the child's thinking has consisted of collecting observations, sensory data and experiences and evaluating them for his preferences and what made him feel best. Abstract thinking now joins in. Abstract thinking is having the ability to think of things in the mind without connection to a concrete physical thing or an external sensory experience. It is creating ideas solely and independently in the mind. This is possible because of a powerful step in language and cognitive skills. The child has formed the ability to separate a word from its physical counterpart. He can think of it using only a word, rather than needing to physically touch, see or sense it. This is the start of abstract thinking.

The direct experience of the world changes as the child can consider abstract ideas about the world, opening the way to create connections between his experiences. This is creative logic based on abstract thought. With the maturation of the brain at this age, the child can formulate ideas and concepts based on analysis and thought from the raw materials of observation.

Developing abstract thinking moves him from his subjective world to an objective one; from a self-oriented world to one including others. He moves from his previously yin state of receptivity to a yang state of outward focus. He is fully able to make decisions, taking great strides forward in self-sufficiency, individuality and autonomy. His main models shift away from parents to society. From the extensive fund of experiences, observations and sensory data, he continues to build logical concepts and enters more fully into the adult world. Physical growth continues throughout the middle to late childhood years.

The child can now enjoy the playground of his logical mind and its creative concepts. Abstract thought requires a creative mind proficient in imagination. With their roots firmly and deeply anchored in creativity and imagination, abstract thinking and logic argument will eventually have precedence over pure experience. Logic without creativity is like an adding machine but logic founded on creativity leads to originality, innovation, invention and advancement and individuality. One imitates, the other invents. One works with what is; the other creates what will be.

Age 11 to 14 – integrating
Global consciousness

All advancements initiated in the ages seven to eleven are further developed, perfected and integrated into the child's interactions with the world. He can act on the structure of his own thinking. With a shift to a greater objectivity, his use and understanding of abstract and logical thinking slowly develops based on the concrete thought and facility for imagination before it. Think of this process as the brainstem providing letters and the midbrain and limbic system contributing words to enable his cerebrum to build sentences, paragraphs and whole books.

Much of this phase is involved in preparing the child for the next important and enormous surge of brain growth, mental and physical development and life change – puberty. Puberty marks the end of childhood and is the entrance portal to the full adult world. He will move beyond the brain into the mind and higher abstractions as he becomes fully creative, including the ultimate creativity of reproduction.

Revisiting the question What is childhood?

At the beginning of this chapter the question was posed, 'What is childhood?' Now that various aspects of a child's life and development have been elaborated, it might be time to reassess that question. Childhood is evidently a time of enormous transition. From a fixed physical concrete world to a fluid creative mental world, a child learns to shift his consciousness, ever flowering and expanding. He sequentially identifies and incorporates each stage of growth before he moves to the next. The child starts with the concrete physical reality of the first year of life, then forms his own individual reality through emotions, judgment and choices and finally experiences the flexibility and creativity with abstract thought and logic. His world continues to enlarge with ever expanding capacities – physical, emotional and mental. Correct development creates objectivity that incorporates previous information in proper perspective. At the end of childhood development, he is ready to embark on the exploration of the subtle creative mind. He has grown from the concrete to the abstract; from dependent helplessness to self-awareness and personal identity.

The ideal situation for the child is one in which the normal stages of mental and physical development are allowed to unfold in their own way. There is a time for the enactment of each stage. Most of all, the best thing is to step into the children's world and experience their life through their perspective, by their rules and their logic. For parents, this perspective will allow them to provide their child with the balance of natural unfolding, and appropriate stimulation as well as gentle direction, guidance and constraint. For homeopaths, this understanding and perception of the child will give a more accurate perspective of how the child experiences life and what should be happening at what time. When the natural progress is disturbed and at what developmental stage will be more easily recognised with this understanding, facilitating the prescribing of an effective remedy.

References

1   Hahnemann S. Organon of the Rational Art of Healing. Dresden: Arnold, 1810.
2   Adler M. Mortimer Adler Quotes, Think exist website. Available online at http://tinyurl.com/ylobkfu (Accessed 16th December 2009)
3   Maslow A. Brainy Quotes Available online at http://tinyurl.com/dp68w (Accessed 16th December 2009)
4   Franklin B. Wikiquote Available on line at http://tinyurl.com/c6vel (Accessed 16th December 2009)
5   Van Zandvoort R. The Complete Repertory 2005 in the Reference Works Computer Program, San Rafael CA, Kent Homeopathic Associates.

6   Ballantyne J.W. An Introduction to the Diseases of Infancy, Edinburgh: Oliver and Boyd 1891.

7   Phelps W.L. Creative quotations from WL Phelps Available online at http://tinyurl.com/yebq74r (Accessed 16th December 2009)

8   Descartes R. Discours de la méthode pour bien conduire sa raison, et chercher la vérité dans les sciences (Discourse on the Method of Rightly Conducting One's Reason and of Seeking Truth in the Sciences) (Part iv) Leiden. 1637.

9   LeBoyer F. Pour Une Naissance Sans Violence. Paris. Éditions du Seuil, 1974.

10 Santayana G. Dialogues in Limbo. London: Constable and Co. 1925; New York: Scribner's 1926. Quotation available on line at Quotations by George Santayana http://tinyurl.com/fgftt (Accessed 16th December 2009)

5

METHODS AND TECHNIQUES

Some basic principles and ideas about source-based prescribing uses were discussed in chapter three. Chapter four has given details about childhood development and stages of growth. Starting from this foundation, this chapter will elaborate about the methods of perceiving, interviewing and analysing information from the patient.

The source is the simillimum; the first end point of the journey with the patient. With source-based prescribing, homeopaths investigate the world of the source energy in patients. There is no one method to do this. There are only principles upon which each homeopath develops his or her own style.

Here are some hints and suggestions to assist in learning more about this method as it applies to children, and as a foundation for developing a personal style.

The child-centred view

Successful source-based prescribing naturally depends on skilful and accurate case taking. The only way to accomplish this is to look at the world from the patient's point of view - the child's view. During the entire interview, case management and all times in between, you must step into the patient's world, leaving your world with all your ideas, analysis, interpretations and experiences completely behind. You become the 'unprejudiced observer' of which Hahnemann spoke. You are going on a journey to a place you have not been before, with the patient, in this case the child, as your host and guide. We must have the skills to perceive what the child is experiencing from his perspective, with his language and choice of expression. By looking at the world through the children's eyes, we come closer to perceiving how they are experiencing their world. It is in their personal experience that we will find the specific characteristics of the source altering their healthy state. Observe everything with wonder and acceptance as the reality of that world. Accept and be with it.

It is not enough for you to step into his world asking your questions and making your observations. You have to go one step further, setting aside your adult thoughts, concepts, analytical ability and experiences and completely accept the child's reality. This concept and what needs to be done is built on the differences of the child's way of thinking and experiencing from adults. Suffice it to say, the more the homeopath can follow in the mental footsteps of his child patient, the more accurately he will perceive the source in the case. Keep this in mind with each case example. You will be able to experience how the homeopath is allowing the child to show the direction the interview should take, through his movements, actions, facial expressions, interaction with others in the room and his symptoms.

Looking at the world from the patient's perception is not limited to children. It is the key to source-based prescribing for adults too. In fact, proficiency doing this for adults will make treating children that much easier and conversely, developing these skills while treating children will open up more possibilities for your adult patients. More will be said about this important point in chapter six.

Following the leader

Homeopaths have all been trained to use their intelligence, analytical minds, memory and experience to solve their cases. Yet now the very last thing you want to do is try to make logical sense of what you are hearing. As automatic and tempting as that may be, it should not be done. That would be pulling the patient's world into yours, evaluating it by your standards. Remember, you have left your world and are experiencing the patient's world. He is the expert; only he knows what is reality; only he is living the energy of the source. It does not matter if their inner experience makes sense to you or not. To be successful you must step into his worldview and accept it as true for him. Follow his lead. Go where he takes you.

Compared to traditional methods, this 'going with the flow' method of case taking seems far too unstructured and unfocused ever to result in collecting enough pertinent information. On first being introduced to these ideas, many homeopaths worry that they would end up lost in a morass of irrelevant, unrelated details. That can happen but only if the homeopath is not paying attention and understanding what is happening. You must follow the patient's lead, but equally important is that you also pay close attention to everything that is happening, with the confidence that you know where you want to end – at the source.

I recall an experience similar to this I had while travelling in India. While visiting Mumbai, I was told of a place well worth seeing. The Banganga, a very large spring-fed water tank and temple built in 1127, is one of Mumbai's oldest surviving structures. I hired a taxi to take me to this unique site. The taxi went deeper and deeper into the crowded recesses of the city, until the roads were so narrow and winding, we could barely pass unscathed. The dwellings became smaller and more rustic. With each corner we passed, I became more perplexed about where the driver was taking me. Surely, such a significant, popular and sizable heritage site would not be located here where everything was so crowded. There were barely any signs of city life. The surroundings just did not match what I had expected to see. I had relied on the taxi driver to know how to get there. Where was I going? Just as I was feeling completely and irrevocably lost, the taxi could go no further and the driver motioned for me to get out and walk. Where in the world was I? I walked just a few meters, and suddenly I was at the top of the Banganga, its magnificent expanse of water opening up before me. It seemed to come out of nowhere and certainly where I had least expected it.

How many times before and since I have experienced the same when conducting a patient interview with these methods. It is in the nature of following the patient's route through their world that the homeopath might feel lost, disoriented, perplexed and without normal landmarks. These feelings are more pronounced if the homeopath is trying to make sense of what he is hearing, or rectify the patient's experience with what is 'normal'. On the other hand, if the homeopath is an unprejudiced observer, along for the interesting journey, without concern about symptoms, remedies and prescribing, then it is possible to explore the source energy with curiosity and wonder. Then suddenly, often when he least expects it, everything connects together and the source appears.

Confidence in the process

How is it possible to just let the patient meander where he wants to go, talk about anything that crosses his mind and still end up arriving at the source? The simple, encompassing answer is that you must have confidence in the process. You know that the patient is in a specific state, that the source energy is the font from which everything springs, especially all the peculiar symptoms. Furthermore you know that the patient has no choice but to manifest the exact constellation of symptoms from the source that will reveal its identity to you. When you truly understand these facts, you know that it is inevitable that the patient will demonstrate the remedy he needs. Rather than approaching the patient with apprehension about 'finding' the remedy, you can relax in the knowledge that the remedy will display itself to you.

While enjoying the journey to the patient's inner world, you must also stay alert to observe where you are going. Never forget where you want to end up; the patient shows you the route to get there. The surest way to stay on the direct path to the source, is to stay attentive to the peculiar symptoms. When a patient brings one of those to your attention, you follow it along. It is not too directive to ask the patient to elaborate more about a particular symptom or statement they have made. Those are the signposts along the way, indicating that you are on the right track. You can gently encourage or nudge them along by enquiring more about the peculiar things they say.

Often it seems as if the patient talks about diverse, unrelated topics or brings up irrelevant details. From the homeopaths' view, the information may seem extraneous and unrelated to the main symptoms or issues at hand. Rest assured, connections are there even if you cannot perceive them. All aspects of every part of a patient's life, experience, symptoms and events are interrelated. It is far more fruitful to approach the patient knowing everything is connected and have the patient keep elaborating and describing until he has brought out those connections for us to perceive.

As mentioned above, you do not want to analyse or use your mind to rectify what the patient says with your knowledge and experiences. By doing so, the patient's experience becomes trimmed and modified in your mind until it resembles what you know and what you are familiar with. The analytical mind filters out anything that does not fit into its constructs. Then you no longer have the patient's true experience: it has become your version of what you thought he said filtered through what you accept as possible.

What versus why

Our analytic mind responds to the question 'why' because it is best at explaining, theorising, speculating and pursuing discourse and debate. Generally there is not much value found in either the homeopath's or the patient's speculation why he is the way he is. Hahnemann clearly warns about the futility of pursuing the 'why' of any medical situation. He advises not '. . . to weave systems from fancy ideas and hypothesis about the inner nature of the vital process and origins of disease . . .' or '. . . to try to endlessly explain disease phenomena and their proximal causes . . .' To understand a patient the homeopath wants to perceive what the patient experiences. The question is, 'What is your experience?' Answering 'what' requires a description, not an explanation. A description is the undisputable truth of his reality as he lives it. The source is revealed by *what* the patient experiences, not *why* it came to be.

One aspect of case taking that is different between children and adults has to do with the active mind. From the previous chapters, you know that children have far less analytic abilities than adults. They do not yet have that equipment fully functioning. The process of maturing includes the development of getting the analytical mind up and running the show. For the homeopath's purposes, that is a big advantage a child has over an adult patient. It is not necessary to spend as much time and effort getting them to set aside their fertile mind and the fruits of its analytical functions. Their daily lives have to do with what they experience and not with why they are experiencing something.

The movement conversation

As was discussed at length in chapter four, children learn, communicate and interact with their world in a more tactile, sensory way than adults. Therefore, they are much more likely to have significant movements displaying their state. Usually, the child does not suppress his movement impulses. Responding to what you observe in the child is like having a conversation with the child. He moves as his part of the conversation and the homeopath replies. Understanding that for a child movement is communication helps see the child's behaviour in an entirely different light. The child is not just randomly moving, wriggling or being restless. Each movement is a statement from his source.

Watch the 'movement conversation' between the mother and the child, or between yourself and the child. Observe what is peculiar or out of ordinary about a movement. You will read in Dr. Anand's case of the child with coeliac disease (see chapter seven, case 7.1) how the child loved to climb. It was peculiar that he had no fear of heights. Also he moved in circles, another peculiar symptom. Both were significant to the choice of remedy.

To have a conversation with a pre-verbal child, observe and ask about what you see. You will be amazed to realise that the child frequently responds to your questions with more or different movements. Though he does not speak with words, he will speak with motion.

Chief complaint

Where would a homeopath be without some symptoms to investigate? They are the link between the patient's state of being and the substance that will relieve them of their suffering. They are all we have to determine a patient's remedy. Homeopathy's view of symptoms is much different than in other fields of medicine. There are more kinds of feelings, sensations, difficulties and thoughts that are symptoms in our eyes than even the patient's themselves. Homeopathy uses a finer mesh in the screen that sifts through a patient's experience of himself and his life to gather up all these valuable bits of information. Despite all the care and attention to detail, there is even more information that is available from the patient when the metaphorical, symbolic and holographic nature of aspects of a person, including their symptoms is considered and appreciated.

With this perspective, a vast amount of valuable symptoms can be used that would otherwise pass by us undetected as the homeopath speeds his way through a patient's story to the more obvious, familiar, yet limited information.

Since all symptoms, actions, thoughts and characteristics emanate from the inner state, investigation of any one of them will lead the homeopath to that inner state or source. You could start the case anywhere, knowing full well that you will always end up at your destination. If you are travelling from Rome to London, you could travel over Europe by car, around the Mediterranean and Atlantic Ocean by ship, you could walk or you could fly east through the Middle East, China, Pacific Ocean, North America and the Atlantic Ocean. Each route gets you to London. Barring a leisurely, meandering vacation route, most travel by taking the most efficient path. So it is with case taking.

What is likely to be the most efficient path to the source? Following the patient's lead serves well to get to the source. To do so, you must recognise when the patient is opening a door for you to walk through. An obvious entry point is displayed by the patient; it is his chief complaint. By definition, it is what is bothering him the most. The chief complaint is the place where the body has chosen to focus its most intense energy, making it a most fruitful place to look for information. Within the chief complaint, you often find enough peculiar and distinctive symptoms on which to choose a good remedy. An adult will confirm what is bothering him the most. For a young child, it is often what the mother experiences as bothering her about the child the most that will be deemed the chief complaint. In any case, this is a great place to start the case. If the mother's concerns are actually springing from her own state and not the child's, it does not matter. The child's state will always be revealed to the unprejudiced, discriminating perceiver.

The chief complaint is not the only place to find useful information. Any symptoms from any part of the patient come from the inner state, and therefore can be helpful. When there is a stress on the patient, their inner state becomes more active, producing additional symptoms usually not seen when their life is quiescent. Therefore a time of stress will often reveal clues otherwise compensated for or not present. For a child, these times include teething, weaning, mother returning to work regularly, starting school or daycare or the birth of another child in the family. It is often helpful to ask what happened during these kinds of events in the past.

Staying peculiar

At the very heart of homeopathy is the concept of regarding every person as a whole, individual, unique being with thoughts, physiology, reactions, ideas and a personality distinctive to them. Individuality has always been central to homeopathic prescribing and it is even more accentuated now. Rather than focusing on common, generalised characteristics to categorise children into one of several known types (see chapter two), their distinctive, individual features are emphasised and utilised for prescribing.

The goal is to perceive the source: the starting point can be the chief complaint. Regardless of what entry point is taken, the real aim is to identify any peculiar symptom. What is rightly perceived as peculiar designates the path to deeper awareness of the source expressing itself. Staying on that path, with meticulously precise awareness, without getting distracted by the various byways from the patient's plethora of information, is essential to success. The objective is to find the simillimum – the source. This can only be achieved by keeping an unprejudiced focus on the aspects of the patient that are the source expressing and calling attention to itself – the peculiar, unusual and strange.

If a traveller in Germany, aiming to see the Glockenspiel at München's Rathaus suddenly sees that all the signs are in French, it is likely he has strayed from the desired path. He must return to a place where the signs are once again in German. So it is with homeopathy; out of all the information given to you, stay only with that which is peculiar and unexpected. Otherwise you might meander for hours in a realm which has no possibility of leading you to your goal.

Attention must always be kept focussed on the peculiar to remain on a course leading to the source. The peculiar symptoms are the source expressing its own state of consciousness, far from the human world and human experience. That is the world of the illogical, unexpected, fantastic and unusual. It is the world out of this world and into another.

Any expression is only peculiar in the context of being present in a human being. The energy or consciousness expressing itself through its own structure is not peculiar at all. In its own natural state, that energy rightly expresses itself as one particular substance; it is the source of that substance. The energy of a daisy existing in the world as a daisy is normal for it in that structure. The energy of the daisy trying to express itself through the structure of a human does not work. The attempts are experienced as symptoms and classified as the peculiar and strange. The daisy energy needs to be removed from the human being. Any energy expressing itself in its own natural structure is normal, not peculiar. Only in the context of a human being, does this energy become out of place, producing peculiar manifestations.

Experiencing life of the source

A homeopath approaches the patient with the knowledge that they are living, in part, the life experience of whatever energy has sequestered itself in their normal energy field. It is his task to identify that energy. When he does, it is called 'the source' and the prescription is based on that.

Living as he does from the dictates of whatever energy field is active in him, the patient is not consciously aware that there is an interfering energy altering his normal human life. Though he may certainly be aware when he does not feel well, has symptoms or is ill, he is rarely fully aware of the difference between his normal human energy field and his current one responsible for his ailments.

A person involuntarily expresses what his energy state instructs. The peculiar symptoms coming from the source, coalesce to give a distinct pattern of some other energy field. If the source energy is of an animal such as a mammal, spider, snake or bird, these characteristics will be seen. The same is true if the energy is from the plant or mineral worlds. The patient is living life with some other consciousness, be it a structure, organism or creature. The person sitting in the clinic in front of you looks like a normal human being, yet you know that their life is complicated by the life force of some non-human energy.

In T. H. White's rendition of the King Arthur and Camelot fables entitled *The Once and Future King*,[1] there is a masterful section which describes the experience of living as another creature. As a child the future King Arthur grows up in an adopted family, completely unaware of his real parentage or destiny. He is befriended by the magician Merlin, under whose tutelage he is given an eclectic education that will serve him well in his later years. Arthur's school years are more fun and exciting than the average classes, as seems to be the case whenever magic is involved. To understand birds, Merlin turns Arthur into a bird; to learn about fish, he must live as a fish. Merlin puts Arthur in the state of being of those creatures to experience their life to the fullest. This is the closest I have ever found in fiction to describing a proving. Reading these chapters of *The Once and Future King* gives the perspective of a source energy inhabiting a person's energy field and rendering him like that substance. Arthur is still himself, but he is also the bird or fish, compelled to live the life they have. How much more vivid is the experience and understanding of a source or substance when a person has lived it from the level of their energy state. This is the basis of our provings, and also the basis of source-based prescribing.

The patient experiences the same thing; living some other substance's life all the while living in a human world and doing the best he can to maintain his human existence. He will be partially living as a bird or fish, or any one of the millions of other creatures, plants, substances or energies in the world, just as Arthur did for that short while that the magic lasted. The opposite occurs with homeopathy's magic. Rather than allowing him to experience that foreign energy, homeopathy releases him from experiencing it.

Each time homeopaths sit in front of a patient, they are in the presence of some substance's energy masquerading in its human guise. How intriguing!

Working in my clinic, I often ask myself, 'What is presenting itself to me today? Will the patient be living in the shadow of an animal, with plant energy or the structure of a mineral leading his life? Will I learn what it is like to live the life of a papaya, an artichoke, a jumping spider, a lizard, some phosphorus, a palm tree, a rose bush, an ox or an iron compound? Which one of the millions and millions of substances on earth, each of which has its own unique energy expression, will I get to know today?'

I am reminded of the former Microsoft advertising tag line 'Where do you want to go today?' As I face each patient, to me it reads, 'Where will I be going today?' Which of the breathtaking varieties, complex and innovative survival strategies or aspect of awe-inspiring inventiveness of the Universe will I have the privilege to glimpse into today? Patients hold the answer; it is their life.

Patient undivided attention

You know your goal, you know how to stay on the road to your goal using peculiar symptoms as guideposts. How do you take the first step? How can you approach the child patient in such a way that he feels comfortable enough to allow you to walk with them on this journey to the source? In this regard, using source-based methods are not different than other homeopathic methods. A trusting, safe, comfortable rapport with the child is essential.

Depending on the nature of the child, he or she may feel some degree of shyness, apprehension, excitement, openness, fright, irritability, reticence, ease or friendliness. Of course, the whole process of acclimating to you and the situation reveals useful information. From whatever starting point, you must build a trusting, comfortable rapport with the child. Up to the age of about three to four years old, I recommend including the parents during the entire interview. Once the child is verbal, if at all possible, I recommend talking with the child without the parents' participation. Often children of this age are accustomed to attending pre-school or daycare, making the parents' absence a familiar occurrence. In my office the wall between the consulting room and the reception and waiting area is made of glass. Serving as a giant window, it allows the parents to visibly witness the child at all times. Additionally, the child knows he can see the parents at any time.

There is a practical reason for interacting with the child on his or her own. The homeopath's goal is to create a safe, neutral environment in which the patient can venture into the world of the source – a world of irrational, weird, bizarre, odd sensations, thoughts and feelings. This can be very different than the parents' typical way of interacting with their child. When their child complains of a monster under the bed, parents usually discourage him from these thoughts, often presenting the logic of the situation. Parents intervene with logic or behaviour correction if the child has an imaginary friend, is frightened that the parents are leaving him, wants to tear apart his toys, or other manifestations of an imaginary world. And rightly so! However, for purpose of homeopathy, the child's imaginary world is of central importance. You want to hear all about it, in all its fantastic, illogical, strange and peculiar splendour. A parent sitting by in the interview of their child cannot help doing what they usually do – influencing, correcting or discouraging these fantasy illusions.

The exception is the child's playtime. Within some broad parameters, generally parents let children play uninfluenced and undeterred. Playtime is a sanctioned time for the child to display all their imaginary ideas, fears, creativity and peculiar symptoms. The source is where children go when they play.

How it works

Encouraging a child to play, draw or tell a story is to give permission for the child to be himself, in his natural state. Homeopaths are sincerely interested in what the child has to say, what he imagines, how he sees the world and how he experiences it without any correction, reprimand or alteration. Listen to the child with patient, undivided attention and genuine interest. Rarely is anyone listened to so intently, thoroughly and with such open acceptance. That alone is amazingly encouraging. Given such attention, children love to tell their story and share their world.

Now that some of the basic ideas and methods of source-based prescribing have been outlined, the next step is to look at a case (case 5.1) and see these ideas in action.

Case 5.1   Asthma

Patient
A nine-year-old girl (NN) with allergies and asthma

Consultation
Mother's story
I started by hearing the mother's description of the problem as she saw it. Her information is objective and conventional, reporting the typical diagnoses and treatments that have been tried. She is not able to tell us anything about her daughter's inner feelings and experiences. In fact, as

with most parents, it does not even occur to her that the inner imaginary world of her daughter has anything to do with her current medical problems. Later it is evident how different the mother's logical, adult view is from the way the girl experiences her problem.

M: My daughter has had a stuffy nose for a year. Since then she had three colds at different times. Recently she got a cold and then got better for a week then she got sick again. That scared me. The first cold was regular without a fever but she had a hard cough and stuffy nose, even more than her normal. When she got sick the second time she got a fever. I took care of her with natural things like herbs and oils at night to breathe. I have been thinking she has an allergy. We had an allergist test her and she does not have allergies in a big way. The doctor said that she might possibly have a slight allergy to dogs. We have two dogs and two cats. I cleaned her room from top to bottom and now we don't let the dogs inside the house but she still gets sick.

The doctor also said that she is getting asthma. We gave her inhaler treatments for two weeks but nothing changed. The nose congestion is the same. We went to another doctor and tested her all over again. There were no allergies showing up on these tests. That can't be right. I see her nose is congested and she is coughing all the time. I know something is wrong. We tried three different nasal sprays, which the doctors changed every seven days. We irrigated her nose with salt water. I continued to give her herbs. Still, she got sick twice during that time. The last time she had a high fever of 106 deg. F and the doctor said she had a slight pneumonia. He gave her antibiotics for five days and she got better. Something is still there. You can hear her with her stuffy nose and cough.

The day after the antibiotics she went to school for the first time. She went into a nervous breakdown, with screaming and yelling. She did not want to be there. She is our only child. She is a very mature girl but she gets upset very often. Whatever bothers her, she talks about it and lets us know.

My pregnancy was smooth, natural and normal. I was very happy. I run a movie production company and worked the whole time that I was pregnant. We were shooting a movie and the filming lasted a year in a foreign country. The first three months my stomach got very upset with nausea and morning sickness. I was always dizzy and did not feel well. She was born on her due date. The delivery was perfect.

As a baby, everything was great with her. I was so happy and so was she. The first three years she got one cold with a slight fever once a year and that was it. She had her immunisations. When she was four, she got scarlet fever. It was so bad with that terrible sore throat, rash and high fever. I was very scared. From then until the present, she gets colds a few times a year. When she was seven, she got mononucleosis with a fever of 104. Her throat was very red and she had large lumps in her neck.

She is smart and that means a lot. She does not talk very much. You have to pull the words out especially if she is trying to analyse something. She speaks a lot when she is happy and excited or when she is upset. When things are not the way she expected, she gets upset. She has a strong character and is very decisive. She knows exactly what she wants. When she likes something, she really likes it. When she doesn't like something, she doesn't. She is a very good student and organised.

She puts her heart into having a good relationship with her friends. Recently she was depressed because she was having problems with some friends. Two of her best friends moved. She thought that they were her friends and that they loved her but then they moved away. It really affected her. She is very artistic and likes writing stories.

Patient's story
Now it is time to hear from the patient. The girl is poised, pleasant and at ease in the consulting room. Despite the mother's warning that she did not like to talk much, she was open, communicative and verbal. For children over age six, I frequently start by asking what is their understanding of why they have come to the doctor's office. This question serves several purposes. The first is to establish from the very beginning that I am interested in their opinions and point of view. Additionally, I get an idea of how much the parent has informed or involved the child in his own health.

Dr: Do you know why you are here?
NN: I came because of my cough and stuffy nose.
Dr: Tell me about this.
NN: Sometimes it comes out when I try to blow my nose. Other times it gets stuffy and I can't get anything out. It usually happens that I can't breathe through my nose. It gets blocked. I try to breathe in and ohhh it is stopped. If I really breathe hard it goes into my mouth and I spit out phlegm. When I cough it is deep. I get a tickle in the throat and I have to cough a lot. It happens especially when I am running and exercising but it also happens a lot at any time. When I breathe a lot, I start coughing. It gets loose and I produce mucus. It is light green or yellow green. If I blow my nose sometimes there is blood coming out. One night I woke up and I

couldn't breathe because the cough was so strong. I felt scared. I started crying and that made it worse.

Comment NN is comfortable and open, easily talking and giving her symptoms. There is nothing peculiar in the description of the cold and cough until the very end. The coughing makes her scared. This is the hint pointing the way to follow. Interestingly, her cough made her mother scared too.

Dr: In what way was it scary?
NN: I was so scared. I feel all closed in and closed up. I felt like my body was separate from the outside. When I breathe I feel I am attached to the world. I breathe in air and it is part of the world. The inside of the body has its own air and then it starts getting dirty. Since I can't breathe in with the world, I feel I am separate. My air is separated. There is a block from the cough.

Comment Have you ever heard anyone describe a cough this way? Very quickly, NN is in her private world of her own individualised experience. It only took three questions to get here, following what is peculiar. From a general cough, she has taken us to the sensations of closed in, separated, attached, dirty and blocked. To feel closed in is to be separated. To breathe is to feel attached, not separated. Any of these would be worthwhile following, but I pick just one for now. I will remember the others to follow later, if they have not come back spontaneously in her conversation. By the end of our interview, each and every one of those peculiar words will be connected to her inner state.

Dr: Tell me about the block.
NN: The block happens when the cough is there. It is like the phlegm and the cough are mixed. I need to get it out. If I get it out by coughing, then I can't breathe in. If I have phlegm or the cough, it doesn't want to get out. I keep coughing and coughing. When I cough, I start the brick to come out.

Comment The cough is the effort to get it out past the block. The block turns into a brick. The brick is now the most peculiar.

Dr: Tell me about the brick.
NN: The brick is there. It makes the tickle in the throat. There is a line right here in the throat. (She gestures to her throat.) I can feel something there. It tickles. I feel it going around the neck. When I feel that, I have to cough. When I cough, I get it out and after that I feel it again. It comes back out.

Dr: This is very interesting. Tell me more about all of this.

NN: I am separate from the bottom of my head and mouth here and the body (She points to her throat again.)

Comment By asking about the brick, she brings up the idea of separation again. What is the connection between a brick and separation? I don't know, but she does. Listening carefully and patiently, she will tell me.

NN: When I breathe in the mouth, I can't breathe into the body because there is something stuck right at the neck. It is the brick. It feels like a big one here. (She points to her throat again.) There is a big red brick here. It is spinning around. It is rectangular. I have to get all the air out. It is something mean and stops the air from coming in. Sometimes it stands straight and the air comes in the sides. That is when it spins around and stops the air.

Comment Does any of this make sense? At this point, it doesn't. I know I am on the right track if things don't make sense to me because that means I am in her world. She has told me about coughing, separation, a rectangular red brick that spins, and the air getting stopped. It is a credit to how comfortable she feels that she is so forthcoming with these descriptions that make no sense to the adult, logical world. She and I both know logically there is no brick, but she experiences a brick in her throat. I will explore this with her. She describes the brick stopping her air and being mean. 'Mean' is a new word. What does it have to do with a brick? In the world of logic – nothing. That is what makes the statement peculiar and worth following.

Dr: Tell about it being mean.

NN: It is mean because it doesn't want any air to get into my body. If it was nice, it would stop spinning or help the air come in. Since it is mean, it stays there and makes it harder to breathe. The cough hurts sometimes because it is pushing so hard to get the thing out of me.

Comment Her actual experience is becoming clearer. I am not asking why she feels this way or why is the brick there. I am only interested in what she is experiencing. I am very curious about this spinning brick in her throat.

Dr: Tell me more about it being mean.

NN: It is so mean because it wants me not to breathe so I would get scared. It wants me to be scared. I get so scared. (She holds her hand at her throat.) It is moving around. Something inside my head is spinning around with the brick. It is in motion and moving. The block is hypnotising me. I have to cough. When I spit phlegm out I feel normal again. The brick is spinning and I am hypnotised and spinning around. It is just the head spinning. The brick is nice to my other part down here (She points to her chest.) There is dirt there. It likes dirty. When I am spinning I want to fall down. I am going to pass out. I want to go down and cover myself. Something scary is coming. It is like thunder everywhere.

Comment She brings back another word, 'dirty', that she initially mentioned. It hardly matters which peculiar word I would have chosen to enter into her world because once in, all the words will show up and be connected. It is interesting to note that her reaction to being scared is to cover herself.

Dr: Tell me more about being scared.
NN: I am scared because someone is coming. You know, like when a bad person is coming to kill you. They are going to do something bad and hurt you. They are coming and I hear footsteps. Everything is so scary. They are about to turn the doorknob and it is so scary. What can I do? It stops and then it is not spinning. I still want to get it out but it still blocks most of the air. I can get some air. But the brick is there and I can only get in a little at a time.

Comment Scared is the feeling associated with coughing and the mean, spinning brick. Being scared is also associated with someone coming to hurt or kill her. That is not so peculiar. It is more usual to be scared about a person coming after you. Then, quite spontaneously, she leaves the usual and goes back to the peculiar; the spinning brick. During the interview, a patient often leaves the peculiar, returning to something sounding more normal. As they hear themselves talk about these unusual, weird and illogical things coming from their inner state, they feel odd and retreat to the commonplace. It is our task to gently guide them back to their inner state. Here she spontaneously goes back into her inner state and I did not have to do anything to encourage her.

Dr: This is all very interesting. Can you tell more about all of this?
NN: It is nice to the bottom part. It blocks the air from coming in. It keeps collecting dust and stays dirty. The brick likes it being dirty and not clean. It is trying to make the upper part dirty by spinning.

Comment She is clearly in her imaginary, inner world; the world of the source. I have no idea what is going on. I don't understand about the dirty and clean and the brick and the upper part and the spinning and the block. I am content just giving her free reign to tell me all about the truth of her experience. I have full confidence that if I am patient and listen to all she tells me, all will be revealed in the end.

Dr: Tell me more about this dirt and being dirty.
NN: The brick likes it dirty. When it is dirty, I feel like I have to cough. Dust is there. A lot of people cough with dust. There is dust everywhere and I have to cough and sneeze. It feels all like gross and sticky and dirty. It makes me feel dirty. I have to put water in there so I drink water. This dirty feeling is just like I went into mud and got all covered with dirt. I have to clean it and take a shower. But the dirt is inside and I can't clean it. I try to drink water to rinse everything out. Water can't get into the body because of the brick. The brick suctions the water like a sponge. It sucks out most of the water. Water cleans a lot out but it keeps building up dirt again. Water gets it out and then it comes again. It gets dirty over and over again.

The brick suctions like a sponge but it is hard, not soft like a sponge. For some reason I can get food in with no problem. It is the water that is a problem. Water could clean out everything if the brick was not there and all water could get in. I want the brick out. Then all the dirt would leave and I would be fine. The brick makes the dirt come again by blocking the air.

I have energy when I am clean on the inside. I am new and fresh. When I am sick, I feel more dirty. I get a sick feeling when I am dirty. When I am clean I feel totally energised. That is how I feel after drinking water. Then ten minutes later I feel dirty again. When I am sick I get a double effect. I already have some of the dirty feeling and then I get sick and that makes me feel more dirty. After being sick when I get better, I feel really clean. The clean feeling lasts two days and then the dirty feeling comes again.

Comment Isn't this interesting? I am getting a better idea of exactly how she experiences her cough and asthma. Sickness is associated with the sensation of dirty or clean. The presence of the brick keeps her insides dirty, making it hard to breathe. The brick is of central importance.

It is common that people with cough or shortness of breathe drink water to ameliorate their symptoms. There are several dozen remedies listed in the various rubrics about cough being helped by drinking. Should

I consider any of those rubrics? Spongia figures prominently, which is fascinating in light of the fact that she mentions the brick is like a sponge. Is this Spongia? It is far too early to think and analyse, or even consult rubrics because I have not yet heard all that she has to say about her experience. If the brick is a sponge, she will take me there.

Dr: Tell me about the brick.

NN: I am not sure what the brick is but it makes me feel scared and shivering. It is hard and sucks up a lot of stuff including water but not food. It doesn't suck up dirt if I ever get dirt into my body. It is fire engine red and scratchy and hard. It has something like suction from little tiny holes and that makes it scratchy like a hard carpet or rough wall or even a brick. I can feel the little edges of the holes. Those scratchy edges will cut my fingers.

Comment Now the brick does not sound like a sponge. She has emphasised the dirt and dust, so I will follow her.

Dr: Tell more about the dirty feeling.

NN: If I looked inside I would see all the sticky, mushy mud covering my body up to the neck. The head is clean. When it is medium it doesn't feel sticky like gooey mud, it just feels like dirt. It feels worse when it sticks stuff together. The insides are all weird and mixed up. The insides are spinning and they go every which way. Some parts are supposed to be over here but they are mixed up with the parts over here. (She points to her head and then to her chest.) Everything in the body is covered in dirt. It is a weird feeling as if the body is like a mansion that has not been touched for a long while and had gathered dust. No one wants to enter it because it is scary and dirty and musty. Part of the air is scared away and does not want to come in. When the air enters, it blows all the dust away and the brick suctions it all up. Sometimes the suctioning is good but then the brick gets the dust stuck to it. Some goes away when air or water comes there but a lot stays there feeling dirty and old and scary. It is a haunted house. The outside looks nice and pretty but when you go inside everything is covered in dust and dirt. Everything in there makes you cough and sneeze. Everything is sticky and muddy and mixed up. I can't get it out.

Comment Recall that she initially mentioned being scared because the cough could not get out. Here again, she mentions 'can't get out'. This connects the dirt with the cough and the cough with getting it out.

Dr: Tell me about getting it out.

NN: The first thing is that you have to cough. Everything is covered and sticky. It can also be dirty and dry. The throat is dirty and is not connected to the lower body because of the brick. On the bottom it feels wet and mushy and muddy. Everything sticks to it. If the brick were not there, the dry head part would mix with it and everything would become regular. The down part is too wet and up is too dry. The brick is pushing everything away. It all slides away. When something is in the throat or head, it all slides away. I feel that when stuff goes to the edge of the throat. It gets pushed away. If you put something on it, it slides off. It is dry and you can't really breathe. There is no moist air because the brick blocks that. The brick likes the wet, cold, dirty place. The head is clean and dry and not sticky.

Dr: Tell me more about the wet, cold, dirty place.

NN: It is like a humid sticky place, a humid jungle with big ponds where the floor is muddy and icky. Inside me is cold even if it is humid. The desert is dry and nothing is there, not even dirt. It is clean. It is hot up here and down is cold (She points to her head and then her chest.)

Comment Slowly, she is clarifying her experience. I want her to continue.

Dr: Tell me more about the hot and cold.

NN: There is dry and clean and hot which is up in my head. That is like the desert. There is wet and dirty and cold which is the humid jungle. That is the down part. The brick separates them. If they mixed, they would a perfect mixture of warm and soft

Comment Her experience of life is one in which a brick separates the perfect place of warm and soft into two areas: one is dry, hot and clean, the other is wet, cold and dirty. Water and air, which could clean the dirt, are not allowed to pass because the brick blocks the way. Coughing pushes against the brick to get it out so the two sides can blend again. This is her world.

I have heard about the separation and its characteristics, but now she has introduced the idea of the perfect place – warm and soft. I will follow her and find out more.

Dr: Tell me about warm and soft.

NN: Warm and soft is when you stay in a room and like it. All around the walls are a sponge. Everything is soft and if you fall, you have a nice warm soft place. It is so soft like pillows on a bed or a rose. You can rub your cheek to a rose petal or fur or silk and fall asleep. A sponge is soft. You feel welcome in a space like that. The weather is warm. It does not give you shivers and you are not sweating. It is the perfect temperature. It is a welcoming place. You can just fall back into the soft sponge walls and be welcome.

Comment The sponge is of less importance than the concept of a soft, welcoming place. To her a sponge means soft, nothing more. If the brick was gone her world would be warm, soft and welcoming rather than what it is to her now – dirty, scary, closed in and separated. She has introduced a new idea – being welcome. In what way does it fit in with everything she has told me so far?

Dr: What does being welcomed feel like?
NN: The brick is not soft. It is hard and scratchy with pointy edges and dirt. The mansion is not welcoming at all. You get a dirty feeling if you go into a mansion. It is like rolling in mud. There is not much air and you can't breathe. It has not been cleaned and everywhere there is the dust like my insides. It feels it can't breathe because the dust is going everywhere. There is no window open and no air can get there. It is closed up like the brick. You can't breathe since the air is dusty and dirty. It makes you cough and sneeze. You have a scary feeling.

Comment Notice that when I ask about feeling welcome, she answers by describing a place not welcoming at all, using all the words and concepts she has brought up so far – hard, scratchy, dirty, can't breathe, no air, closed up and scary. This is her world as she experiences it day to day. She feels not welcome, and that is what she can most readily describe. She personifies the mansion, 'it feels it can't breathe' and equates it to her own body. She is the mansion, and everything she says about it, is true about her.

NN: You are spinning because you can't breathe. Everything is dirty and not one thing is clean. Dust is on the floor. Your finger gets dirty if you touch anything. If you fall on the floor it would hurt. A sponge floor would be soft. If you don't watch out, you could bang your head. The brick is like a wall and it blocks. It has to spin. It has to be a rectangular wall and not a circular wall. I am glad it is not a brick that is a circle otherwise I couldn't breathe at all.

The mansion might be like that. When people get scared from some-thing inside the mansion like a ghost they want to leave. They can't because the windows and doors are locked. Everything is closed up. Dust gathers. The inside is connected to dust but not to the outside. That is like my inside. If one window is left open some air can get in.

Comment This is the second time she has brought into the conversation the phrase 'closed up' she mentioned initially. She is spontaneously connecting all the seemingly diverse words and concepts together. Even though a lot of the pieces are becoming connected, I still do not fully understand her. I don't know where she is going. I have no idea about a remedy. All I know so far is that there is an upper and a lower part separated by a mean, red, rough brick that spins keeping the dirt below and preventing air and water from getting past it. She longs for a soft, clean, sponge-like welcoming world that would not hurt her, even if she fell. To find out more, I shall follow her lead and ask about the term she brought up.

Dr: Describe closed up.
NN: Closed up is when you staple or nail wood to the door. If a mansion got closed up all the stuff of wood or metal just slams down on the whole place. Sometimes they do that at zoos to get ready for animals. You have to come in and clean once in a while just so it doesn't get dirty. The problem with me is that the brick never goes away. Everything is closed up and slammed shut. If you are inside, you can't get out. The outside can't get in. The person inside is closed up. There are so many walls - wall after wall surrounding that place and that person. If you break through one, there is another one. You get really tired after a while trying to break through.

Comment From the very start, she mentioned 'can't get out' when describing her nose congestion. This links her physical problems to the sensation 'closed up and can't get out' of her inner state. When this correlation is present, we are definitely on the right path to the source.

NN: Anyone closed in won't be able to breathe. Right after being slammed shut, you can breathe but after a small while, like a week, they would start to not breathe. There would be coughing and probably their head is spinning. You feel like falling in a sponge place. If you felt like that you can fall. But when you are closed in then you only fall in a hard place and it would hurt.

Comment When she is sick and can't breathe, she would like to be in a soft, welcoming place. Instead, she is in a hard, hurtful place.

NN: In a sponge place, the room is soft but you are still closed in. It is better there because you can fall and feel fine. When you are closed in a bad place you are going to die. You are stuck in there and can't get out. You feel like you must run to all the doors and try to open them or break through one of the walls. If you couldn't break through the first, then try the second one. Outside you would have utensils to help you but you are inside closed in and you can't get out. You feel scared and lonely. You have to break through if there are a lot of walls around. You hammer for a long time until the walls will break open and have broken through. You would go over into the dramatic. I would faint before I would stop breathing. I mean over dramatic because it would start when I knew I would die. I would cry and cry and if I cried I would cough more and then the brick spins and the head spins.

Comment For the first time in these passages she describes the reaction she experiences to being closed in – a desperate, dramatic urgent need to break out. Sankaran classifies this type of reaction as tubercular. Whatever circumstances, sensation or perception initiates or causes this reaction, its desperate, urgent need to get or break out places the patient's state in a group united by a tubercular theme, or miasm. Sankaran's designation and methodology of miasms is beyond the scope of this part of the book, and will be touched on later. Suffice it to say now, her reaction indicates a tubercular miasm, serving to start the identification of the remedy's qualities.

All along, she has clearly and with confidence described how she feels and experiences her state. This is not unusual with children. Given a safe, trusting environment, they often are able to relate their perspective very well. They are far more comfortable with the illogical and fantastic than we are! The other area that will reveal information about their state are the dreams. Often their dream life is not that much different from what they experience in their waking life, but there can be additional subtle clues.

Dr: What dreams have you had?
NN: I had a dream about two dead bodies. I was in an elevator with two friends. There were silver doors and we couldn't get out of the elevator. We couldn't open the door. There was a hook into the elevator that was holding it over a fiery place. We were stuck inside the elevator. Someone from the outside world opened the door. When the silver doors finally opened there were dead bodies. I saw the dead body and screamed and covered my face. He told us to jump out and land outside. One person missed and fell into a fiery place. When he fell I screamed too. I had the feeling that I wanted

to scream and cover myself up and stay in my own little world. I wanted to go to a happy place.

Comment She has mentioned wanting to cover herself up before when describing the mean brick and being scared. Covering herself up is the way to enter into her own world, her own happy place. In the dream she is closed in a small place. If she tries to leave, there is danger, fire and dead bodies. She becomes frightened and screams, possibly similar to the screaming she did when her mother first took her to school. As before, being scared, she covers up and retreats to her own little world. I want to know more about this happy place.

Dr: Tell me more about going to a happy place.
NN: If something bad happens, I feel that I want to go away to bed. I go under my arms and image something else like sunshine and trees and oxygen and good animals. It feels like I am in my own perfect world. Nothing can go wrong. There is no fire and no bad things. When I uncover, I go back to the real world which is bad.
Dr: Bad means what?
NN: Bad is at that point where there was fire and people were dying. If you stay awake you would be stuck in that world but if you make it up, then you are in a better world. When you are down there everyone around is screaming and dying. There is fire everywhere with lots of red colour. I imagine red is a really bad colour. If you break the roof or a wall or a brick you are going between the lower world and higher world. If you make it up to the higher world it is nice with trees and flowers, like my own world. If you looked back down you have memory of the lower world and that is scary. There is fire and dying. I don't like when people die and I don't like fire or being near fire. It makes me cough. You have to break through and push up through the bad, push past the block between the good and bad worlds. Even if you get up to the better world, the bad world is still there. It should get mixed with the good world to become good. That is like breaking my brick. Anyone living down there in the bad world would want to break through the brick.

If you are stuck somewhere, you have to push up the wall to break out. It feels like pushing up at something blocking. It is bad when it is blocking something better. Pushing it up feels like a victory because you have finally broken that thing that was separating you.

I would rather be in the higher part than the lower part. My head is better then. The higher world is clean but it is still too dry and hot. That is a problem. The bottom part has everything wrong with it; there is nothing good about it. Lower world is more icky and gross and sticky and mushy. Usually lower is bad and higher is good.

The lower world is bad. You are stuck down in the lower world, left behind and you can't get out. All you see is fire and red and people falling and screaming and running. The king of the lower world wants everything to be bad and stay the same as the lower world. His chair is high up so if anyone tries to escape he can push them down. He is bad and wants everyone to live in misery and die and live in fire and darkness.

NN: The upper world is full of clouds and sunshine and brightness. There is also a big chair but it is not very high. It is soft and cushiony. The whole world is full of softness and clouds and white and blue and trees and grass. You can fly there. The king of the higher world lets everyone be welcome.

Comment The upper place is warm, soft and welcoming. This ties in with her earlier descriptions. In addition, previously she included oxygen as part of the upper world, clearly linked to her breathing troubles.

Dr: Describe being welcome.

NN: Welcome is when they are not kicked out. They are treated with care, given a bed and food. It is better if the two worlds join so that everything is good. My own little world is like the upper world, especially because it doesn't seem real. It seems like a better place than the world. My own little world is more real. I go there when I am scared and when I don't like being in the real world. I am only scared of the real world because it has fire, killing, falling, being left behind. It is a dirty place and you can get closed in. If I don't like it, I leave. I like being in the upper because you are always welcome. It is not like when you are left out or left behind. Then you are sad and scared and lonely.

Dr: What happens to a person who is left out or left behind?

NN: If you are left out you feel sick. It is really, really bad if you go home to your house and your parents say that they don't want you there. You start crying a lot because you feel that your parents don't love you. You feel sick inside, your stomach hurts and you get headache. You feel very lonely. No one loves them in the whole world. Parents usually are happy and love their kid. Your parents are the number one that love you but if they don't, then no one can love you. You don't have a home because your parents didn't let you go there. You are very, very sad and angry.

Comment Everything connects up now and I have a complete picture. She has clearly and directly explained what life is like for her. There is a lower place that is bad and a higher place that is good. Her body manifests her concept of this separation by being divided into lower that is wet, cold and dirty like a jungle and the upper part, which is dry, hot and clean like the desert. The separation prevents air and water from passing, thereby produces the cough and asthma, her physical complaints. The brick blocks the passage and to get to the upper good part, she must break through the brick. She told us that the brick is mean because it wants to keep the dirt in the lower place. Here too she describes the king of the lower place that wants to keep everything bad. She is stuck in the lower place, left behind all alone by those she loves, closed in and she can't get out. It is dirty and dusty and she can't breathe and she can't get out. She tries desperately to get out, hammering against the walls, but it doesn't work. She is stuck there. She is so scared that she cries, screams and gets dramatic but that does not help either, in fact it makes things worse. Instead, faced with this scary situation, she covers herself up and goes into her own perfect world where it is warm, soft, clean and comfortable, full of trees, air, clouds, sunshine and brightness. It is an ideal place where she is taken care of and never left behind, where she will never be separated. It is a place where she can breathe.

What is the symbol of what she experiences day to day? What is the hub of all her symptoms? The brick. The brick creates the separation, the division of the two worlds; upper and lower. The brick keeps everything dirty, causing coughing and won't let air in causing asthma. The brick is hard, rough, hurtful and cuts, the very opposite of her ideal, soft, spongy world. The brick prevents anything from getting out. She can't push through, or break out, therefore she is stuck and closed in all alone, left behind in that dirty, musty, unwelcoming mansion that no one wants to enter. She has told me herself, 'The problem with me is that the brick never goes away.'

Having understood her state, I ask her one final question.

Dr: Do I understand you correctly? Do you want the medicine I give you to get rid of the brick?
NN: Yes! That is it. Get rid of the brick. YES!

Comment I have never run into a more certain confirmation of having taken the right path to the source than the joy expressed on NN's face. Her expression told me that she knew she had been listened to and understood. It is our goal to perceive what needs to be cured from the patient's view. For NN, the goal was to get rid of the brick. It was not to cure the asthma or stop the cough. Those symptoms were not the real problem, they were only the effect of the problem. When I asked her about getting rid of the brick, she knew that I perceived all that needed to be known.

Analysis

This case is here mainly to demonstrate the case-taking method of allowing the patient to go at their own pace and direction. All I did was ask her to elaborate on certain points that I found to be peculiar in her statements. The combination of her lead and my inquires led me into her inner world with ease. Of course, not all cases are as fluid as this one. The methods used, however, are similar in most cases.

Of course, the remedy I prescribed is also important and I will now discuss the analysis of the case. Basically, the information needed has already been noted above. She has a tubercular reaction to her perceived sensation. She is panicked, scared and desperate to break out. What makes her react this way? What is she experiencing that drives her to break out? The answers to these questions will guide us to the family.

She perceives the world as divided into upper and lower parts. She is closed in the lower part where it is dirty, harsh, rough and hurtful. To make matters worse, it is her loved ones that have left her there, scared, alone and dying. Despite her best efforts to break out, she can't do it. She is stuck there. This experience is replicated in the way she experiences her physical symptoms. She also tries to get air through her congested, blocked nose, breathe through the congestion, but is unable to.

She escapes this terrible, scary reality by withdrawing into her own private idyllic fantasy world of softness, care and comfort. The experience that she wants desperately to break out of is one of the separation into upper and lower worlds, where she is confined, closed in, stuck in the lower, awful one. The only way out for her is the fantasy world of her own making where everything is soft, pleasant and welcoming. There is a group of plants that has just these themes, Sankaran's homeopathic family Hamamelidae. Cann. ind. is a well known member of this grouping. Cann. ind.'s fantasy life of vivid illusions, pleasing surroundings and enticing sensations of colour and music serve to escape the monotonous limitation of a boring existence. The similarities are apparent, however for NN, her fantasies of warmth, softness and togetherness serve her to escape the reality of the restriction and confinement being separated from her loved ones.

What is her Catch-22, no-win situation? On one hand she feels confined in the lower place all alone with the mean king in the form of the brick, who blocks the passage and likes the lower world to be dirty. Closed in like that, she is scared and can't breathe. She tries to break out by coughing forcefully enough to get the air and water past the brick, to clean the area and unite the upper and lower worlds, thereby forming the same soft, clean, welcoming world of her fantasy. When she tries this, the brick spins more, filling the place with more and more dirt and dust, exciting her cough, which makes her dizzy and she can't breathe. She is exhausted from the ineffective efforts.

She stops trying, covering her head and going into her fantasy world that is just like the upper world. She doesn't do anything to get out of this horrible scary place and the coughing subsides. She can breathe again – for a while. Unfortunately she isn't really in that wonderful soft upper world. She is still in the lower world, closed in, left out, separate, sad and alone. It seems better being confined in a soft place than a harsh one, but ultimately she is still closed in, the air will run out and she will have to break out. Now it is harder, because she has given up trying. If she does muster the effort to try to break out, she will arouse the dirt and start coughing again. She is stuck in the lower world whichever way she tries to get out: breaking through the brick by coughing or escaping into fantasy. No win: no way out.

Choice of remedy
The only solution is a remedy that will merge the upper and lower worlds, remove the need for fantasy and the desperate acts of coughing. That remedy is in Hamamelidae which reacts in a tubercular way: Juglans cinerea, the butternut. She was given Juglans cinerea 200c.

For those who are not familiar with the ideas and methods of source-based prescribing, botanical family and group characteristics or Dr. Sankaran's miasm designation, the choice of Juglans cinerea may be perplexing. The results clearly reveal that this is a correct remedy for her. Equally clear is that without these new methods, it is very doubtful it would have been chosen. There simply is not enough information about Juglans cinerea from the traditional sources to highlight this remedy. It is listed for the following rubrics:

- RESPIRATION; Difficult
- NOSE; Coryza
- GENERALITIES; Faintness

These rubrics would hardly have been enough to definitively point to that correct remedy. Most of the other rubrics or materia medica references are general or local symptoms and not the peculiar, distinctive characteristics on which precise prescribing depends. In addition to demonstrating the case taking method, this case confirms how valuable the new approaches in making a successful prescription.

Follow up – three weeks
Dr: How are you now?
NN: The cough is starting to go away. I have not been coughing. I like flowers and lots of trees. I love fruit trees but I don't like cactus. They have too many spines and spiky sharp things sticking out. When you put your hand at it you get cut with all those pointy things.

Comment Immediately after commenting about her cough, she spontaneously talks about cacti. She is using the same words she used to describe the brick.

NN: I like fruit trees a lot and trees with flowers. I don't like trees with green only; they should have flowers. I do not like pine trees; they have spikes. When you look at them they are pointy at the top. I don't like tall trees. I could never climb up to the top. With other short trees, I can climb them. I like to feel that I can master things. If you have something that is your goal in your mind, after you do that you have mastered it. There is a connection with mastery and the brick in a way. By mastering something, you get rid of it. If I want to master the brick, I could get rid of it.

Comment It is great that she is feeling she can master the brick, as opposed to her previous state where she could not break through or overcome it.

Dr: Describe mastering the brick.
NN: The brick has sections. It is only scratchy on one side – on the side that is facing up. If you could turn it around it would suction up all the dirty stuff. But I don't know how to turn it over. I had a dream. I was at my school with my best friend. It was her birthday. There were older kids there too and we were walking into class. They had water balloons and were throwing them at our heads. I had a hat on and it got all wet. My friend went to get the hose. I knew my mother would get mad since I got wet. I ran into the classroom and we ran around chairs spraying everything with the hose.

Dr: What was the feeling in the dream?
NN: I felt wet and cold. I was scared of the older kids. It was a different kind of wet and cold. In the lower part it isn't wet watery like the dream. The lower part is muddy wet; all muddy and wet and sticky.
Dr: Tell me about liking fruit trees.
NN: I love peach, apricot and apple, plum, orange and grapefruit. I like that they have lots of branches. Nut trees are ok. I do not like almonds but I like peanuts and cashews, walnuts and pistachios.
Dr: (question to the mother) What does she like to eat?
M: She loves nuts. She eats them every chance she gets. She likes these very special pecans, hazelnuts, almonds, cashews and pistachios. She definitely does not like walnuts.

Comment These interesting food preferences never came out in the original interview. Look at the difference between what the mother and the patient say about her preferences for nuts! Though the mother said in the initial interview that the daughter tells her whatever is bothering her and talks freely to her, she does not know her daughter as well as she believes.

NN is clearly better and I will wait and see her again in two more months.

Follow up – three months
Mother's comments
M: She been sick for a year and I have not seen any change. After the first two weeks, her cough disappeared. That is all. She still has a runny and stuffy nose. It is not letting her breathe. She has been sick with fever three times since the last six months. One day she had a fever of 100 deg. F. She was fine after that and but then got sick again with a cold lasting 4 days. There was sneezing but no cough. Today she has a cold and a fever of 101. I brought her in because now the cough has started again.
Dr: Is there anything different about this cold than the colds before she got a remedy?
M: This is the first time in her life she has fever for only one day. Otherwise there are no differences. She has been having nightmares for several days.
Dr: Are there any differences in her at all, in any area of her life, her mood, her sleep or eating?
M: I have noticed that she is more patient now and more willing to cooperate. She is not as frustrated or desperate. I am sure that is just

because she is more mature now. It seems that she is more understanding when she is sick. Before she would get desperate and upset. In general she is better and more mature.

Comment We know from the previous interview that the mother gets very scared when the daughter is ill. This fear is making her emphasise the symptoms and overlook the changes for the better that have taken place. The daughter has no more cough, even when she gets a cold. Previously, her fevers reached 104–105 deg. F, and now they are 100 or 101 deg. F, lasting a much shorter duration. Most of all, she is far more calm and less desperate, indicating a deep, fundamental change in her inner being. The mother is not giving the remedy any credit for this improvement despite these changes having occurred in only the last three months. Of course, the mother doesn't know about the brick! Let's hear what the patient has to say.

Patient's comments
Dr: How are you?
NN: The cough has gone away. My nose is the same and running and stuffy. Even so, it is a little bit better. I am not blowing as much as before. Before I was blowing constantly and now it is only two or three times a day. Also after blowing, it is clear and I can breathe. That never happened before. Then after a while it gets stuffy so I have to blow again.

It feels like the brick went away. That caused the cough. It feels that my insides have cleared. When I breathe in, I can feel it open. It is fresh and clean. Before I could not breathe in deep because of the brick. The brick is completely gone. Now I am sick a little bit but the clean and dirty mixed together and turned everything inside fresh and clean. There is no more muddy dirt. I feel better because the cough is gone and the nose is less stuffy. I am 75% better. Half belongs to the cough, which is all gone, and half was the nose, which is half better. That makes 75%.

I have been getting a rash when I take a shower. It is itching and it turns all red. After the remedy it started happening more often. Every time I take a shower I get a rash on the legs. It is red and bumpy and little bumps and they really itch. After when I scratch it dries and then goes away after 10 minutes. After the remedy, I got a stomach ache. It is stopped now after a week. Every other day I have a strong stomach ache like a cramp. One day I had to come home from school and it lasted all day. It was happening for two weeks and then stopped for a week and then again. Now it is not as intense as before.

I have been getting sad easily and I am suddenly crying. I am not even unhappy. Why am I crying?

Comment Since she asks the question, it is likely she has thought about it and has some ideas. I would like to hear what she has to say, so I turn the question back to her

Dr: What would make a person cry like that?
NN: They would cry if one of their pets is lost or if someone in the family has died. Sometimes I get sad because I am feeling bad for something. One time my mother was talking on the phone. Daddy and I wanted one thing too but she made something else and I didn't want it. I was crying because mother had prepared the whole thing and I didn't want to eat it.
Dr: What did you feel?
NN: I was unhappy. I had a dream in two parts. I was at my house. It was morning and I had just gotten up. The dogs were inside. I went outside and felt that someone was following me. I turned around and there were grey dogs. They looked like coyotes with big bodies and a small head with pointy ears. They were from another world. They were chasing me and I was screaming. I was so scared and I wanted to get out of that feeling. I was running away from something. They grabbed and bit me. I was frightened and screaming. I did not want to be in their world. Every time I have a nightmare, I scream and it is a real scream.

Comment She continues to improve. Her rash started increasing after the remedy, and that is a good sign. Recall that she had scarlet fever at age 4. Though we don't have details of the symptoms, it is highly likely that this rash is the residual of that past problem and will resolve soon. The dream indicates that she needs another dose of the remedy. In it, she is expressing her state – a frightening world that she wants to get out of. I repeated Juglans cin. 200c and had her return in one month.

Follow up – four months
Father's comments
F: A few days ago she felt a bit hot. That is it; she has no other symptoms. Her spirits are great. There is less and less mucus and discharge. This treatment is helping her because she is better and better. There has been a big change from a year ago. She was never cured before.

Patient's comments
Dr: How have you been?
NN: I did get another stomach ache but it was gone right away. There have been fewer rashes and not every time I get a shower. My stuffy nose is the same. Three or four times a day I blow my nose but I can breathe through it just fine. The cough has been gone a long time. I am very happy all the time now. I have been happy every day. When I come home from school I tell my mother and father I am great.
Dr: What about the separation and the brick?
NN: There is no separation between the upper and lower. What brick? Oh yes, the brick. It is all gone. I got a little bit of sneezing last week but this week I am better, completely better. The brick was gone a long time ago and has not come back. My lungs are all clean. The dirt is completely gone from everywhere. I feel just fine.

Comment After hearing so much about the mean brick as the source of her troubles in the initial interview, you can imagine my surprise when, after merely four months, she doesn't even recall the brick! Actually, it should not be that surprising. When the remedy cures, it takes the pathology out of the consciousness. Her failing to remember the brick is the surest sign that her problem is resolved and will stay that way.

More methods

Case taking is not a random process, nor is it a routine of asking a standard set of questions. To be successful, you must always be paying attention to all the forms of communication. You must follow the patient by picking up peculiar words or symptoms, and carefully inquiring about those unusual aspects of the story. You should ask just the right question at just the right time. Through this delicate dance of careful questioning, listening and observing, you can follow the patient deeper into their world of his source. A question asked when the patient is speaking very close to their source will have a different answer than the reply given to the same question asked at the beginning of the interview. In the example above, what started as a cough became a block and then a brick. Staying with the brick it opened up the world of separation, dirty, alone, left behind and attachment, it brought me to the inner world of the source.

As you will see in most of the case examples, much of the interview is for the purpose of information gathering to understand the patients' perspective and experience. Once you have arrived at the source, the remedy should be clear. It is important not to stop there. Make sure that every single peculiar word, symptom, gesture or observation has been so thoroughly investigated that it connects to the source. At this point, it is helpful to ask questions to confirm the remedy. Often I will cycle back and ask about the same key points again to ensure that I understood exactly what the patient meant, and that every point is part of a whole. How often there is one small little symptom or word that I have let slide out of my awareness because it has not been clarified and remains unexplained. Do not let it go unattended! If you do, you are assuming that loose end fits well with everything else you have understood. It could well be that it is the opening to a deeper level of understanding, leading you to an entirely different remedy, that is a far more suitable. Cycle around and back again through each and every point until you are satisfied they all reach the source.

Reference

1   White T.H. Once and Future King. (The Berkley Medallion Edition) New York: The Berkley Publishing Corporation, 1966.

6

THE SOURCE REVEALED

What does saying that the goal is to 'get to the source' mean exactly? How will you know when you have arrived? Some have misunderstood the source-base method to mean that if a patient mentions that he likes daffodils, he needs to have the remedy Narcissus, or if he says he watches movies about whale migration, he needs the remedy Ambra grisea. Nothing could be further from the truth. As with most misconceptions, there is a tiny kernel of truth buried in there. It is true that source-based prescribing uses all information about a patient, including what aspect of nature he likes and which movies, books and TV programmes he watches. However, the journey hardly ends there. A person is far more than his reading list or floral preferences. Every detail about the person must be part of an overall integrated whole.

Furthermore, these comments are often superficial, requiring intensive investigation to find the core of what is being expressed. For any individual person, an attraction to whale migration could just as easily signify the love of swimming, the need for freedom of movement, the feeling of being small and insignificant or even the need for independence from one's family. In fact, it could mean anything! Only the patient knows what inner state is being displayed outwardly in the guise of the attraction to whales. Source-based prescribing involves taking nothing for granted, making no assumptions and then going to the depth of each and every point until the unifying context is revealed. That is the source.

It has been previously stated that the patient will reveal the source. That is true, however, it is not usually the case that the patient actually names the source. A Lac caninum patient will not necessarily talk about dogs. A sulphur patient will rarely mention sulphur by name. A Nux moschata patient is unlikely to say 'I am like a nutmeg.' Although it is far more common for patients in an animal state to describe and mention that animal by name, source-based prescribing is not dependent on that happening. In fact, getting specific animal or plant names is more often misleading than helpful. Not every person who says they like cats, requires Lac felinum, not every person who is afraid of snakes will end up with a remedy from that zoological group. Whenever a specific substance, animal or plant is named, it is vital to explore what it means to the patient. Remember, you are stepping into their world, so it could mean anything. Approach each word from the stance that you do not know anything until the patient tells you!

Source words

Case 6.1 Source words

I recall the case of a young man who was passionate about baseball. There was nothing else on his mind or of any importance to him. Whatever subject we started speaking about – foods, schooling, friends, childhood, dreams, family – we always ended up talking about baseball. It is a very good thing that our materia medica does not include potentised baseball, for surely I would have been tempted to use it.

On deeper investigation, he revealed that what he liked the very most about the game was the speed of the ball. That key opened a hidden door into his inner state. The issue of speed led on to the topic of competition about who was fastest, who was the winner and who were the losers, how important it was to always improve your speed. The culmination of many other new clues was his statement, 'Only the very fastest runner survives.' It seems there had been a cheetah on the ball field! He never mentioned the animal by name, but when exploring the issue of speed, he journeyed to the source and used cheetah source words.

In an interview (consultation) as the patient becomes more and more connected to the source, he will speak from that perspective. Words, images and sensations directly connected to that source will be expressed. These 'source words' reveal the source. Sometimes that can include saying the exact name of the source, sometimes it does not. Source words include those words reflecting the source's family grouping, characteristics of the source's life in nature, qualities the source exhibits and any other aspect of the source's experience of its life.

It is the homeopath's task to allow the patient to become connected to his source, then recognise when source words are being used and perceive the source from those words. With some patients there is a distinct demarcation when going from the conversation about the normal, day-to-day life, symptoms, treatments, activities and thoughts to the inner world of the source. Sometimes quite suddenly the patient will change the tone of voice, pace of speaking, body posture and language. It is as if you were listening to the Rolling Stones on the radio and then the dial is turned and you are now hearing Chopin. It is the same radio, but everything has changed.

Recall the case of NN from chapter five. The girl went so quickly into her inner state, almost immediately using source words; her transition was not pronounced. In fact it was barely noticeable. To get the impression of this contrast, compare the tone, content and pace of the mother's story with the girl's: they are from two entirely different worlds.

As has been discussed, the patient is living, in part, from the inner state of the source. Any particular source will be revealed through the symptoms, actions and words of the patient. Therefore, the expression of the source will be limited by the vocabulary, age and life experience of the patient. Even with adults, these limitations still apply. Adult patients needing remedies from well-known animals often do name the source. Knowledge of animals is quite common. Familiarity with botany and chemistry, however, is exceedingly uncommon. Consequently, rarely, if ever, do patients give the names of specific plants and almost never have I heard of a mineral named when the source is from those kingdoms. With children, whose range of words and experiences are even less developed, you might expect that it is even more of a consideration.

A collegiate dictionary contains approximately 200,000 words, yet the average adult in America has a vocabulary of less than 700 words. Without extraordinary effort or intentional study, this seems to be all that a child can expect to obtain for daily use. Those few words are unlikely to encompass the rich variety of human experience. Whether adult or child, a patient filters his experience through the only words he has at his disposal to symbolise what he is really trying to express. While these kinds of limitations are true in theory, in practice that does not prove to be a problem using source-based prescribing.

The name of the source is only one word out of many words, images and sensations emanating from the source. To prescribe a specific source, it is vital to have a whole constellation of words and sensations, all interconnected. The name alone would not be enough. I had a case on this point. The girl's favourite animal was a dolphin, and she talked about them extensively. On deeper examination, however, none of the other source words connected to dolphins. They all pointed to macaw, which I gave her with great result. It is likely she did not know there was such an animal as a macaw, however, she was familiar with dolphins. Therefore, she ascribed the qualities, sensation and experiences of her source on to what was known to her – the dolphin. My job was to see past the dolphin as a symbol of her source and find the real source. That is your job too.

The power of names

The actual name of any source is our descriptive addition to the energy of the source; a symbolic shorthand for it. Our propensity to name things started a very long time ago. According to the first book of the Bible, Genesis, no sooner is Adam up and ready for his day, does he find himself naming 'all the beasts of the field and fowl of the air'. With hearty abandon, we have been naming things ever since. Carolus Linnaeus (1707–1778) organised the naming system of the entire world of living organisms, self-proclaiming that he was, 'carrying on what Adam had started'. Much of the structure he established is the basis for what is used today and many of the names he assigned to plants and animals are still familiar to us.

The miraculous human facility for spoken language bursts on the scene at about the age of one year. As any parent will confirm, once started, the child literally has a vocabulary explosion, acquiring words and the names for things at an astounding rate. It is possible to witness the child experiencing the exhilarating power of naming; associating a word to a thing, creating a symbol for it. And what a powerful and essential capacity it is! Deprived of naming means being denied connection to the human community. To employ this vast aptitude is to enrich oneself beyond measure.

There is a hauntingly powerful scene demonstrating this in the motion picture, *The Miracle Worker* (United Artists, 1962) which is the story of Helen Keller. Blind and deaf from infancy, she is imprisoned in her dark and silent world. When Helen is about seven years old, a teacher, Annie Sullivan, is hired for the monumental task of teaching her. After difficulties almost beyond endurance, there is a breakthrough, stunningly portrayed by actress Patty Duke as Helen. The miracle is a moment of naming. Helen names water by connecting the symbols she feels in one hand to the fluid flowing over the other. Once the power of naming has been restored to her, she instantly perceives its significance. Experiencing her own vocabulary explosion, she dashes around the front garden, pointing to an object excitedly demanding the name, just as any child does who has discovered the power of words. Though her language is not heard but felt, the process is identical.

Words as symbols

The name of a substance is a verbal, written, or as in Helen's case, tactile symbol for the actual thing. We have created a whole world of such symbols. Our thoughts, words, deeds and ideas come to us as symbols, are expressed to others as symbols and are understood only as translated from one symbol to another. Similarly, we can hardly talk about symbols, since we are also floating in a world of nothing else. We do not just live in a world of symbols; we live in a world of our own individual symbols of our own making. Communication consists of each of us trying to find a place for our world of symbols in the context of someone else's world of symbols.

Expressing individuality

There is always a delicate balance between the personal meaning of the words someone uses and the need to communicate that meaning to another, which build the bonds of relationships, families and society. As much anyone tries to comply with standardised meaning, he is always using his own dictionary, his own meanings from his own world, whether he realises it or not. Involuntarily and inevitability, he relies on his personalised meanings of the symbols he uses. Nutritionists say we are what we eat: I say we are what we speak.

When I say 'lion', you know to what I am referring. But do you? With each word I use, I am taking a draught from the deep well of my own personal reservoir of symbols and meanings. To facilitate communication, each person agrees to forgo some of his individuality by using systematised and standardised meanings of these symbols called words. In daily life, communication would come to a stand-still if each word required elaboration and description about the nuance of individual experience. The dictionary is the guide to agreed standard meanings and the uses of these symbols. The dictionary ignores individualisation and leans towards the homogenisation of meaning for the purpose of communication. Allopathic medicine does this too. When a patient is given a diagnosis, he is, in essence, told what symbol he represents irrespective of his individualised symptoms, experiences, modalities, emotions, memories or feelings. His personal meaning for his illness is of no consequence at all as he is homogenised into a universal symbol of a diagnosis category.

Although the ability to make symbols, name things and use standard word definitions is indispensable, there can be too much of a good thing. It appears that in the excited flurry of naming, people often forget that the name is only a representation, not the real thing.

According to Polish–American philosopher and scientist Alfred Korzybski (1879-1950) *The map is not the territory*.[1] The diagnosis is not the illness, not the meaning, not the person's individual experience of the world. Homeopaths skip the map and go directly to the actual territory. We strive to understand exactly who the patient is and how he looks at the world, how he experiences the world. We look out from his eyes, and see what he sees. We ask ourselves, 'What is the patient's unique symbolic use of these words meaning to him?' We step into the world of his symbols, eventually matching it to the world of symbols we use, called remedies.

This concept is not new. The philosophic movement of the 1800s called the 'Romantics' was the first to hold a view that may seem all too obvious today. They said that all art is a symbolic language addressed to a deeper, unconscious awareness in the human soul. Even Freudian psychology nearly 70 years later, with its stress on what is most irrational in man and in its dependence on symbols, is largely indebted to the German Romantics of the same era. Freud's groundbreaking work relied on the then novel idea that humans use symbols in every area of their life. People turn what they see and experience into symbols and then turn their reactions to those symbols into more symbols. He postulated that every part of human behaviour could be understood as logical if we perceived the meaning of a patient's symbols to him. Freud gets the credit for this although Hahnemann preceded him by nearly a century.

Remedy as a symbol

Each remedy is a symbol for a state of being. That symbol speaks in many different languages. Just as a dictionary is a translator of symbols, so is the repertory. The repertory translates the language and symbols of the body, mind and thoughts of a patient into our symbols, the remedies. Homeopaths all have 'jobs at the biologic United Nations, translating the language of the skin, liver, head, lungs, joints, dreams, mind, emotions, thoughts, sensations and experiences and all the others into what is the universal language of the remedy. If a person feels stabbed, the pain will be stabbing. If a person feels nervous, the autonomic nervous system will activate and give out the evidence by moist palms, jittery stomach or shortness of breath. Each rubric and modality, each physical symptom is a symbol telling us what the patients experience in life and how they look at the world.

Many areas of medicine and psychotherapy use the idea of symbols and acknowledge that the body is a symbolic expression of the person. Yet despite this good start, many lose the trail here. They proceed to assign and standardise biologic meanings; a sore throat means the patient does not want to talk: teeth problems always have to do with aggression; cancer is always unexpressed emotion; menstrual pain always means the patient does not like being female. The patient can look up their symptom and instantly be told what it means. There is no individuality here!

There are 2830 species within the Rosaceae family and over 5000 different varieties in just one of those species – the Rose. There are 7200 different varieties of apples. There are 40,000 species of spiders. Of course it is possible there would be more than one source of a sore throat! The repertory lists 339 remedies for throat pain. 339 known homeopathic symbols coinciding with the symbol of the sore throat. I suspect even that number is not complete. Each person's sore throat is a symbol for him, as an individual and we can only find out its meaning from him. One such recipe-style book entitled *The healing power of illness: The meaning of symptoms and how to interpret them* is 270 pages.[2] I just cannot understand that. How long does it take to say, 'Ask the patient'?

This brings us back to the key feature, the essence, of symbols – individuality. The essence of a human being is our individuality, from our fingerprint, to our DNA, to our face, to our thoughts, to our symbols, to the source we are expressing. The essence of homeopathy is the respect, actually the glorification, of that individuality. Step into your patient's world and you will be able to experience who that individual is by reaching the source. The symbols, peculiar symptoms and source words give us the passport to make that journey.

Case 6.2   Naming the source

The next case, presented by Dr. Sunil Anand and reproduced with his kind permission, demonstrates an instance in which the patient names his source.

As mentioned previously, it is not just this that indicates the remedy. The other sensations, feelings and expressions of the patient connect together with the named source to form the totality. Dr. Sunil Anand's case also demonstrates the positive role of homeopathy even in genetic and metabolic diseases.

Patient

The patient is a 14-year-old boy. This case is fascinating because the boy has a serious inherited metabolic disease, Wilson's disease. The basic pathology is a disorder of copper metabolism resulting in the accumulation of copper in the liver but eventually collecting in other organs of the body, particularly the brain, eyes, and kidneys. The excessive copper in the liver causes acute or chronic inflammation of the liver, severe liver disease and a progressive loss of liver function and cirrhosis with the associated elevation of liver enzymes and jaundice. A variety of neurological symptoms are also common. The initial approach in treating Wilson's disease is the removal of excessive copper with chelating agents. Naturally, a diet low in copper is essential. Foods such as cocoa, chocolate, liver, mushrooms, nuts, and shellfish must be avoided.

Consultation
Patient's story
Dr: Tell me your problems in detail.
Pt: I feel very tired. I feel very sleepy. I also have a lot of tension from studies.
Dr: Tell me about each of these in further details.

Pt: Besides the above, the tension often leads to headaches.
Dr: Say more about this . . .

Observation There were long pauses before each answer.

Pt: It's a feverish feeling all the time.
Dr: Say more about this feverish feeling.
Pt: As if there is a lot of heat inside, but from outside my body feels cold on touch.
Dr: Anything more about the feverish feeling?
Pt: No.
Dr: Say a bit more about the tiredness.
Pt: I don't feel like doing anything. I just want to sit in one place without doing anything.
Dr: Tell about the sleepiness?
Pt: All the time. Even now while talking with you I feel like sleeping.
Dr: Now say more about the headache.
Pt: It is on the top of the head and above my eyes.
Dr: What is the pain like?
Pt: It is like a banging.
Dr: Describe the banging a bit more.
Pt: All I can say is that it happens only when I am tense.
Dr: What is tension? How do you experience tension? When do you experience tension?
Pt: It is mainly related to my studies.
Dr: Tell more about the tension related to studies.
Pt: If there is a lot of homework and I have not been able to complete it. Things like that make me tense.
Dr: In what way?
Pt: Then I don't feel like attending school
Dr: Tell more about that.
Pt: The teacher may beat me or punish me.
Dr: Has that ever happened?
Pt: Never.
Dr: In what way do they punish you?
Pt: They send you out of the class.
Dr: What would that make you feel?
Pt: It would be very insulting.
Dr: What else leaves you feeling insulted?
Pt: When my friends tease me.

Dr: How do they tease you?

Pt: When they say that even though I am in the ninth grade, I cannot hop properly.

Dr: How does that feel when they say that?

Pt: I immediately leave from there. I don't feel like playing with them ever. But very soon I become friends with them again.

Dr: What is the experience and sensation within during such an insult?

Pt: I feel very uneasy from within.

Dr: Say more about this.

Pt: I cannot sit still in one place at that time.

Dr: Why?

Pt: It's a sensation of heat alternating with chill. Even during the heat my body is cold on touch.

Dr: Say more about this.

Pt: It is a similar sensation during an exam.

Dr: Say more.

Pt: It is a headache along with this feverish feeling.

Dr: What about exams make you so tense?

Pt: Will I get good marks?

Dr: What if you don't get good marks?

Pt: I feel very bad. I will work hard the following year to get good marks.

Dr: What is your field of interest.

Pt: Mechanical engineering.

Dr: What about mechanical engineering interests you?

Pt: I like to repair things and also make different things with my Mechano set.

Dr: What are your other interests?

Pt: I like math and playing on the computer. I also like to watch TV and musical shows.

Dr: What else?

Pt: When I grow up I wish to rid India of all its poverty.

Dr: Say more about this.

Pt: I want India to be a rich country.

Dr: Say more.

Pt: I want to get the Koh-i-Noor diamond that the British have stolen from us back to India.

Dr: Tell me more.

Pt: They have robbed and tortured us a lot.

Dr: What else did they do?

Pt: They created partition. They wanted to give Kashmir away to Pakistan too.

Dr: What do you feel about this?

Pt: If they had not divided us, our country would be the fourth largest in the world today. Due to the partition we have become seventh.

Dr: Which is the largest?

Pt: Russia.

Dr: Which is second?

Pt: America.

Dr: Third?

Pt: China then Canada, Brazil, Australia and then us.

Dr: What about Africa?

Pt: That is a continent!

Dr: Your geography is very good. What position do you get in your class results?

Pt: I came third in the ninth. But in the recent unit tests my aggregate was second.

Dr: Are you satisfied with that?

Pt: No. I want to come first.

Dr: Tell me more about that.

Pt: It is difficult to say. I just want to come first and will work very hard for that.

Dr: What steps do you feel can be taken to eradicate poverty in India?

Pt: There should be employment for all and we should control our population.

Dr: Say more about your nature.

Pt: I am easily irritated.

Dr: In what way?

Pt: If others don't listen to me I get very angry.

Dr: Give an example.

Pt: If I want to watch TV and my mother does not allow me to. That makes me angry.

Dr: What do you do when you are angry?

Pt: I throw the sheets and pillows in anger.

Dr: Then what?

Pt: Then I feel calm.

Observation At that point I noticed that he sighed deeply.

Dr: What happened just now? Why did you sigh?

Pt: The tension that I had until now has been released.
Dr: What got released?
Pt: Would the interview go well or not.
Dr: Then why the sigh?
Pt: The interview is going good.
Dr: What happens until then?
Pt: It is like an exam. Until I read the paper, I feel a lot of dryness in the throat.
Dr: Tell about that dryness sensation.
Pt: Until I have read the full paper and realise that I know all the questions, I feel the dryness.
Dr: Say more.
Pt: Once I know that I will be able to answer each and every question, I feel relaxed and then the dryness goes away.

Comment Within the case form given to patients when an appointment is scheduled there is what I call a 'creative page' in which patients are encouraged to do a doodle or a sketch of their liking. At some point of the case, what they had created is probed into. The boy had done a sketch of a temple. This discussion took place while probing into this particular sketch.

Dr: Tell about this sketch.

Observation He draws a sketch of a village with homes. A river is flowing from its source. There is a temple high up on a hill with steps leading to it. Birds are flying in the sky.

Pt: The temple at the top is a Ganpati temple.

Observation The picture shows a river flowing down the mountain where the temple is. The river coming from its source has significance. Later he talks about source and origin and about things that should be returned to their source of origin, like the issue of the diamond mentioned earlier.

Dr: Tell about the Ganpati temple.
Pt: I visit a Ganpati temple every Wednesday as advised by my Guru. I prefer to go when it is not too crowded. I feel irritable and suffocated when it is crowded and people jostle one another. I do not like crowded places.
Dr: Tell me your dreams.

Pt: I am playing with my friends or having a party with them. If I see a horror movie I dream of ghosts. I dream about my exam results. I have a dream about falling down into a deep valley.

Mother's story
Dr: Describe him as a person.
M: He is very helpful to his friends. His friends mean a lot to him. He is very caring towards children with handicaps. He is very rigid about his views. He never owns up to his mistakes, though there is a lot of acceptance about his illness.
Dr: In what way?
M: He does not ask for foods like chocolates that he likes very much but which are not allowed to him due to their high copper content. He feels bad that I too have stopped eating it as he cannot have them. He is very attached to me.
Dr: In what way?
M: Since his diagnosis four years ago, I have taken an indefinite leave from my job. Now I may have to resume after six months. He feels very protected when I am around. He is worried about how he will manage once I resume work. Some acceptance has been coming in of late. He tells me not to worry about his illness. When he was ten years old and diagnosed with Wilson's he told me that 'you are with me and I am with you so we need not worry'. He is very tense about his studies. He has a writing problem and is very slow. He often falls ill before his tests. He crams and mugs up until he knows everything, yet he feels he will forget it all. That has never happened. Before a test, he wakes up very early to study and prepare. He is very good in math but languages are a problem. Since grade seven, he has been writing the same thing on the essay topic called 'My Mother'.

'*She is everything to me*
She works very hard for me
If she was not there, I would not be there.'

He cannot stay alone, even now. Someone must be with him at all times. He often says that when he starts to earn he will get a diamond like the one in the movie, Titanic. He has to do things well. If he has not written something to his satisfaction, he gets angry and tears it up and re-writes it.

Comment This topic about diamonds has come up twice; once about the Koh-i-Noor and once about the one in the Titanic movie. That is peculiar and distinctive. This is worth investigating.

The boy is called in again.

Dr: What can you say about diamonds?
Pt: I like them a lot.
Dr: In what way?

Observation He began to move his feet a lot.

Pt: Diamonds shine. It is unbreakable. They are not found much in India. It is a non-metal but has a lustre. The Koh-i-Noor is the world number one diamond. It is so big and priceless. They are found a lot in Africa, deep among coals.
Dr: What more can you say about diamonds and their structure?
Pt: Would you like me to draw a diamond to explain its structure more clearly?

Comment I encourage him to do so and that is when he does the sketch of the diamond.

Dr. Sunil Anand's analysis
For his age he is very precise about his symptoms. It was very important to him that I understood exactly what he was trying to say, that he clarified each point as clearly as possible. He made a point of ensuring complete clarity, even mentioning it to his mother. This characteristic also appears in that he is very transparent in his views. His striving for perfection is apparent from the diligence he applies to his schoolwork, erasing anything not exactly correct. At times, he is very sharp with his words. He can be hard at times and very difficult to convince if he thinks he is in the right.

He has his plans and life clearly defined. He wants to perform well. Even though he is sure of himself at most times, he questions and doubts himself at the time of any performance, like a test. He tries very hard to overcome his handicap. He is also sensitive to other children who are handicapped. He values the number game. He does not break down when his friends are mean to him. He wants to retain their friendship and goes out of his way to help them. He needs the support of his mother, and is very attached to her.

All these point to a mineral source. A person in a mineral state views his illness as a lack or inadequacy, as he does. The need to be perfect in spite of his handicap further confirms the kingdom. The specific mineral is elucidated by his need to be valued by his peers, family and teachers and his high ambitions. He aims high, wanting to be number one.

He is ready to put in as much hard work towards that as required to achieve that status.

He is very hard on himself, requiring that things should be perfect. He is very sensitive to exploitation. He believes that objects should be returned to their source of origin such as the Koh-i-Noor diamond. He wants India to return to its former glory. These point to a precious mineral source. There are several in the mineral kingdom. There are other clues to indicate which one.

There are strong themes of carbon and the 2nd row. He has a strong attachment with his mother. He is not too sure if he can exist separately without his mother. He demonstrates his strong dependence and attachment to his mother; even repeatedly writing a poem about how he would not exist without her. He wants to be independent, yet he still needs support. At times he wants to assert himself and that makes him defy his mother. He dreams of falling from a height. He feels suffocated in crowded places.

What precious minerals do we find in row two? Through his repeated, energetic talk of diamonds in several different contexts, we are witnessing his connection to his source. He volunteers to draw a diamond, which he does gladly. His mother confirms this connection by saying that diamonds figure a lot in his conversations at home. He wants to study hard so that he can have enough money to buy her a diamond like the one that was in the movie, Titanic. His bond to her is symbolised by his desire to present her with a very large diamond.

Choice of remedy

There are many aspects of his case that link to diamond, beyond his mentioning it by name. For this, we can refer to information from the proving. One issue that was emphasised in his comments as well as his drawing was the whole idea of things that originate from their source. The river he drew was flowing downward from its source. The diamond must also be returned to its source, India. The British took it away and now it should come back. He describes the British actions as stealing and torturing and unjust; all acts of exploitation. Exploitation and greed are two prominent themes. Though it has never happened, he worries that he will get punished and beaten at school. Indeed, he feels his schoolmates tease and insult him. These comments are connections to his view of the British exploitation of India in the past.

Diamonds are clear and the more clear and flawless, the more precious and valuable. As he repeatedly expresses, no fault or flaw is allowed. Absolute precision and clarity is required at all times. He works hard to maintain his personal precision; he wants to be a diamond of great clarity and value, to be the number one, the best and the biggest. In spite of having a deep pathology he still manages to get good grades. It is important to him that his value is noticed among the others. He wants to shine, to be singled out in spite of his medical illness, not because if it.

He is given Adamas in LM dosing. LM 1 was followed by LM 2 after two months in gradual stepping potency. After four months he was on LM 4. LM is a favoured scale in cases with deep pathology and weakened vitality.

Follow up – four months
There has been a significant change. The boy has more enthusiasm. He is not feeling as sleepy. He is responding to questions more fluently, as opposed to his initial interview during which there were long pauses before each answer. He does not get as out of breath after playing. His concentration and memory have increased. He is more hungry and able to digest all foods, and as a result, he has put on weight and height. His acidity has significantly reduced. With such a favorable result, his prescription medication dose was reduced to half.

Follow up – one year
This child's general improvement continues. He is studying hard for his 10th level exams. He can stay alone now, a situation unheard of before. Overall he does not feel as tense. He has good stamina. His growth includes puberty changes. He is no longer constipated and has daily stools. In addition to his remarkable clinical and symptomatic improvement, his pathology reports have improved. His liver enzymes are normal. The urinary copper was within normal range. The ophthalmologist was very encouraged by finding no further presence of the K.F. ring after a slit lamp examination, which was present earlier. The dose of his prescription medication was further reduced.

Further comments on the source

This patient exhibited all of the important themes of Adamas: clarity, shine and sparkle, need for fresh air and suffocation in crowded places, order and precision, hardness, hurried, impatient, exploitation and issues of separation.

The source and the case will now be explored further.

Diamond is a form of carbon, so despite its glamorous, precious and valued existence, the substance still has the themes of row two, and especially its member carbon. Those themes include separation, dependence, attachment and sudden danger. The question is 'can I exist on my own, separated?' Whereas all the remedies in the row grapple with that question, each has a different answer. Going from left to right, the row is the story of the progress from absolute non-separation to complete separation. It has been observed by many homeopaths, including Sankaran, Jayesh Shah, Bhawisha Joshi and Harry van der Zee, that this progression symbolises the stages of birth from stable, unchanging intrauterine life to the dramatic transformation of birth with its final separation by cutting the umbilical cord. Each has written about these ideas in detail in their useful and informative books.

Carbon is the remedy in the middle of the row at the tipping point between staying in the inner, dependent world or embracing the outer, independent world. Will he have the capacity to handle the independence needed in the world? Having this vital reaction or not is the central theme of all carbon remedies. There are many carbons in our materia medica; carbonicum salts, Carbo veg., Petroleum, Adamas, Carbon dioxide, Graphites, Saccharum, Kreosote, the carboneum salts to name a few. Regardless of their individual distinctive qualities, they all share the carbon/row two themes.

Adamas is particularly interesting since so much about its chemistry, history, properties and uses seem far removed from the fetal dependence and separation of row two. From carbon to diamond, from the business end of a pencil to the universally acclaimed, prized and coveted, greedily sought, royal crowned, valuable gem is quite a journey. It is made through the crucible of heat and pressure, just as this patient experienced heat and tension when he was trying to achieve the heights of flawless performance. Yet even at its most elevated and valued, the diamond is still fundamentally carbon. In the proving there are issues of babies needing protection, highlighting the second row themes of separation and danger.

What is the never-ending, no-win dilemma for this boy? Where is he stuck in his development? How does his physical pathology embody his inner state? He feels dependent, unable to exist without his mother. Yet, he is at the stage where he also has the urge to be independent. To be independent, he puts himself under great pressure to do exceedingly well at studies and give flawless performances on all his tests, so he will achieve the top, be the very best, the number one and be singled out for his high value. But if that happens, he will be so valuable that he will get exploited by greedy people who will be mean to him, beat or even torture him while trying to steal his value. He will be all alone, separated, in that dangerous situation, unable to survive. He then yearns to return to his source, his mother. She will protect and ensure his existence, keeping him safe from the dangerous world. Yet that means he is dependent again, unable to exist separated from her.

His physical pathology plays a part in this dilemma. As serious as Wilson's disease is, it is the fever and tension that is most interesting and peculiar. When he is working hard to achieve, he gets these symptoms, thus preventing his full effort and fulfilment of his potential. It is in the nature of Adamas, his nature, that despite these flaws, he still does as much as he can to achieve the heights. The pathology and symptoms serve to prevent him from achieving too much and becoming too independent because of his inner state of fear of the separation and exploitation that would result.

Adamas has changed that for him. He is calmer, developing normally, including becoming an independent young man. He no longer has need of the pathology, and as his pathology reports indicate, this is greatly improved.

Case 6.3   Dreaming of the source

The following is another case in which the patient names the source.

Patient

The female patient has suffered frequent severe headaches since she was six years old. Her initial consultation with me was at age eight. Magnesium phosphoricum worked well for three years to eliminate her problems. After that time, the remedy did not have the same beneficial effect.

Minor headaches began to return, and were unresponsive to additional doses or a change in potency. Her mother informed me that her mood was highly irritable, and the remedy had not been helping. Therefore at age 11, I re-evaluated her case and the salient points are presented below.

Consultation
Patient: The headaches have returned and they really hurt. I am grumpy. I sprained my wrist two years ago and it keeps hurting. There is a sharp pain in the wrist like a knife going through it, stabbing it. Someone is pushing a knife into the skin and pulling it out again.

My nose bothers me the most. It is stuffy and I am having sneezing attacks, which are very embarrassing. I don't like to be embarrassed because people might laugh at you because you say something weird. They laugh at you and it is mean and cruel and socially unacceptable. As if someone has a disease that makes her lose her hair and others think is it is funny, so they laugh at her. It is mean to make you embarrassed in front of your friends.

The Dream
We were in a Victorian house. My brother was there with me and we were dressed up of that time. My brother and his friend dressed as skeletons with masks. We tried to pull off the masks. When we got to the last one we couldn't take it off. They had five masks on each. They were creepy, scary masks with creepy skin and a skull underneath. It was creepy, creepy, creepy! I kept pulling off the masks but there was always another one underneath until I got to the skull. It was like when I eat an artichoke. At the heart, it is small. It was just like eating the artichoke until the heart, which has bristles like a toothbrush. When I got to the skull, it looked like that thing because the skull had bristles too. The top of the mask was pointy like a mountain. It was small at the bottom. They had that one last mask and when I took it off, the head was the same size but it was really scrunched up and when it came back out, it got regular sized again. It was small and then I took off the mask and the head got big. Small and big. The pointy tip was like the tip of a pencil or scissors.

The last mask was pointy and straight up. It was the artichoke heart. When you take off the heart it goes back to an artichoke. You go down in the layers. They are small and then it goes bigger. Small and goes bigger. Like a telescope. If you look from the wrong side of it, the other is bigger.

The small gets bigger. Flowers do that. They go from small to big and go back: blossom to flower to blossom. They have to go through a cycle.

Analysis
The dream was a key ingredient in determining a good remedy. If we try to make logical sense of her dream we would miss the point. It does not make sense. For example, in reality, the tips of the outer leaf-like scales are the sharpest. In her dream, the bristles of the heart are the sharp part. We give up our logical thoughts and assumptions and follow her as she moves to the source. She does a good job of describing what she experiences in the dream. The peeling away of layers in the dream moved to one of the key features of artichoke, the peeling away of successive layers to get to the heart, which is bristling. Further source words are the pointy top part of the mask, easily identified with the top points of the artichoke scales. The words 'layers, bristles, peeling off, tip, blossoms and heart' are all source words. The other key element is how the patient moves so spontaneously from skull to artichoke. The connection is vivid for her. It sounds unlikely and peculiar to us, but that is what makes it so fruitful.

It is also important that the source words connect to her physical pathology. Although headaches and irritability are the main complaints, she barely mentions them. What occupies her attention is her painful wrist. The pain is sharp and stabbing, similar to the pointy bristle of the artichoke like the sharp point of the scissor, which appeared so prominently in her dream. The connection between source and physical symptoms allows me to make the prescription with confidence.

Choice of remedy
In her initial interview three years previously, she mentioned liking artichokes along with pasta, fish, candy, and ham. That is an unusual food desire for an eight-year-old child, but by itself, it was not enough to make a prescription. Now it serves as an interesting confirmation after the fact.

I gave her Cynara scolymus (artichoke) 200c.

Follow up – three weeks
Mother
She had two headaches together a week after the remedy and another a few days ago but none of them were too bad. In general, she is more easy going. She had been in that horrible mood of hers.

Patient
I am feeling good. I slept better. I slept more hours and did not stay up late. I can fall asleep better. I am not yelling at my brother so much when he annoys me. I have not been getting my headaches as much. My wrist is fine. I forgot all about it.

Follow ups summary
Over the next 20 months, she continued to respond extremely well to Cynara scolymus, requiring eight doses of 200 or 1M. Her headaches are essentially nonexistent. Overall she is much easier to get along with and calmer with much less anger and certainly not explosive.

When she requires a dose of Cynara scolymus, she presents with grumpiness, irritability, and moodiness with an increased teasing and purposefully annoying of her siblings. She also gets a headache at those times with her usual modalities of better from firm pressure and hot showers. During the ensuing months she often would have dreams of some kind of embarrassment where everyone was looking at her. The violence and fear in her dreams reduced over time. During one visit she reported that she was afraid of masks because they cover your face and then people don't recognise you. Bad guys use masks so they could stay undercover and not be recognised.

Further comments on the source
Cynara scolymus is a member of the Asteraceae or Compositae family. Asteraceae family is enormous with three main subfamilies, one very small, the Barnadesioideae, and two other larger ones, the Asteroideae and the Cichoriodeae. Asteroideae contains most of the members of this family of which we are familiar; Arnica, Calendula, Eupatorium, and Bellis. The Cichoriodeae includes the thistles and dandelions. This is the branch that Cynara scolymus belongs to, along with Carduus, Taraxacum and Onopordon.

In our materia medica sources of Cynara scolymus, anger and violence are noted, as is sycosis but not much else is known. The sycotic aspect has been very clear, with dreams of embarrassment and the issue of masks hiding and covering up one's face. Masks were a theme even beyond the typical hiding aspect of sycosis. Peeling off the layers of masks was a peculiar feature in the original dream that led to the identification of artichoke.

The bristles, or the sharp, stabbing part, are near the heart, covered up. During a follow up she elucidates the added meaning of the mask. It helps the bad guys stay unrecognised. The many-masked artichoke serves to hide the bristling, sharp heart; it hides the violence; hides the injury.

Case 6.3   Living the source

Not all patients will mention the source by name. NN in chapter 5 did not and the following young man does not either. Whether a patient names his source or not, he is living it every moment. It is through the expression of the source in his life, dreams, actions, thoughts and sensations that we are able to identify it. The following case demonstrates this.

Patient
14-year-old male complains of headaches and allergic rhinitis.

Consultation
Mother's story
My son is an exuberant and intense person. When he gets ideas, he is forceful, adamant and definite about them. I would say he is his own person. He can be opinionated and even bossy at times. He wants to be the boss and to call the shots. On the other hand he cannot stand physical confrontations. He avoids boys that are overtly macho or aggressive. He used to be bullied when he was younger. Maybe that is why he can be devious. He had to find a clever way to avoid the bullies.

He is very particular about his food. He eats the same lunch everyday. He lives in chaos; his room is a complete mess. He has terrible breath and does not seem concerned with his personal hygiene.

He likes being in the limelight. He wants to be the best and to be first. That drive makes him competitive. It bothers him a lot that life is unfair. He demands fairness at every turn. He also gets envious of others, especially when they do better than he does. I have seen him hold a grudge. He really loves animals and has empathy for any animal, especially the small ones.

Patient's story
Pt: I get headaches. I also have allergies that make my nose stuff up and run. I am constantly sneezing. My eyes water and are always bloodshot.

Even my ears itch. The most severe reaction is in the Spring when I am affected by pollen and dust. I have a back problem. I think I am out of alignment. My spine is like an 'S' and that makes my whole body tilted. I don't take change well. I want the same things all the time. I eat the same thing for lunch everyday.

I like to give orders, not follow them. It irritates me when someone does not do what I say. I voice my opinion easily. That is not hard for me. If I say something and I am wrong, I stick to what I said anyway. I guess it is my pride. I am not easily pressed into things that I don't want to do. I feel very strongly about my beliefs. I am against liberal thinking. If someone is married, they should stay married. They should never go against their vows. You shouldn't be hypocritical. It is simple; just do what you say you will do. If you promise something, don't cheat. If someone cheats, they have no integrity, no honour. They are not decent. If I make a promise to do something, I must follow through. I don't believe people should get something for nothing. If they are healthy and can work but don't, they are just lazy. I've worked for what I have and where I am. They haven't worked and they get something for nothing. That really bothers me. It is not fair.

I hold grudges. In 20 years you will get your just desserts. I like revenge. If someone made fun of me I would humiliate him in front of everyone. That would make me feel good unless I saw the look on their face. Then I would feel sick because I had just become as bad as them. I want revenge but then if I take it, I don't feel good. They think you are at the same level as some of those people.

Usually I am not envious but I can get jealous. I am jealous of anyone who gets something better than I do or with better ability than I have. In sports, if someone is better and has more points than I have, I get really angry and jealous. I should have that. I have the ability. If I don't like them to begin with, it is very hard to take. I get angry. I want to choke or hurt someone or something.

I think that I am always late but I like to be the first to get somewhere. My anxiety of being late makes me feel hurried. I get very angry if I am late.

I like all animals. My favourites are cats and dogs even though I am allergic to cats. Animal dander makes me sneeze. I am afraid of big cats like mountain lions and bob cats. I also have a fear of falling, heights and insects. I really hate insects, especially wasps, spiders and earwigs. They make my skin crawl.

I have dreams of things that happen during the day. I also dream of bobcats or mountain lions that attack people. Sometimes they are going to attack me. I have dreams of getting money. I like money. I must have money.

I like to get my own way. I don't want others to tell my what to do. I get really irritated. It makes me feel that they think I am an idiot, incapable of doing it. I can do it for myself. I can figure it out by myself. I have to prove that I am capable, that I am a better person than they are. I get angry with my brother and then I cut him down with my verbal attacks. I really feel like being very aggressive and hitting him.

I am competitive. I get irritated if someone thinks they are better than others. I really hate it if they weren't better but they keep thinking they are. Like if they go around thinking they are cool. I just want to go up to them and say, 'You are an idiot and everyone thinks you are.' I am aggravated when they just keep thinking they are cool. They should not go strutting around, wearing sunglasses. They should tone it down. Don't act like you know everything. I think they must not feel they are cool because they think they have to prove it.

Dr: Tell me about your fear of insects.

Pt: I hate insects. I hate spiders, all arachnids. I hate scorpions. They make my skin crawl. They are disgusting. I get a crawling, itching feeling on my skin.

I like to do my own thing. I don't like to be told what to do. It makes me very irritated. You don't have to tell me what to do. They don't even know that they are talking about. I could just hit them in the face. Why are you making fun of me?

I don't like to be dirty or grimy. I hate filth. I must be clean all the time. I feel disgusting if I get dirty. I must take a shower right away. If I was dirty in public I would be really embarrassed. I must be clean. I think others would look and think, 'that guy is dirty.' I am not like that.

I like routines. I order the same foods. It is hard for me to change or be different. I changed schools and didn't like it. I knew everyone, then suddenly I didn't know anyone. I had to make all new friends and build a reputation. I am nervous meeting new people because you have to say the right thing. You might accidentally give the wrong impression. I am not an idiot. I am not inferior.

Dr: Tell about building a reputation.

Pt: That is what people think of you. If you have a bad reputation, people won't want to be with you. My reputation is good, nice. I don't belittle or criticise. When I am criticised I get embarrassed. I get ticked off and criticise back. They cut me down, then I get angry and want to fight back.

Dr: Embarrassed by what?

Pt: If you know a secret about me and I didn't want people to know and someone told. I would be very embarrassed. They cut me down. I would feel small and I would retaliate. I would find the flaw in them and expose it for revenge.

Dr: Tell me more about the dream of big cats.

Pt: It was a quick dream, lasting only a few seconds. I was feeding the dogs and I heard something. I looked up and saw a mountain lion just as it pounced on me. Suddenly, it was on top of me. There was excitement, but not in a good way. There was great fear. It chewed my face off.

Dr: What did you experience?

Pt: Immediate panic; I was really frightened because it jumped right on me before I could move.

Dr: What other times do you imagine someone would feel that much fear?

Pt: If there was nuclear warfare with atoms bombs. I can see the mushroom clouds.

Dr: What about the situation creates the most fear?

Pt: Because they strike so quickly.

Dr: Have you ever felt that fear in your life?

Pt: Once when I driving along on the freeway. We were switching lanes where two lanes merged. We almost crashed and I was really frightened. My heart jumped into my throat. I felt as if I would have a heart attack.

Analysis

In this case, the patient has not mentioned the source by name. We do have, however, many source words to give us a good idea of how he is living that source energy. In the absence of naming the source, the words of the source guide the way. What is life like to him? What does he experience day by day? What is his inner state? How does he see and react to the world?

The crux of the matter is that he is terrified that at any moment sudden death is coming to him. As he goes to school, plays sports, is driven along the road – in every circumstance, every moment of his life, he feels this way. How do we know that? In his dreams, he is frightened when a mountain lion jumps on him, attacking without warning. A nuclear war, the lion, in the car on the freeway – each instance is characterised by the advent of sudden attack, pouncing, death coming fast and unexpected. He has no time to react before it is all over. His heart jumps to his throat. He is terrified, not just at the moment, by in anticipation of the possibility of a sudden deadly attack. His symbol for his fear of sudden death is having a heart attack; again the themes of sudden, unexpected and deadly.

He also lives a life of competition and comparison. He wants to be the boss, in charge and be the best and first. If someone tells him what to do, he feels put down, like an idiot and small. He wants to be the big man, though he feels so small. He freely discusses his jealousy of anyone who is better than he is or has something more than he does. He feels less than others, that they laugh at him and cut him down. He was bullied and humiliated by others bigger and more powerful than he was. He hates hypocrites, cheaters and unfairness. That tells us he also has that tendency. His mother mentioned that he could be devious.

When he sees those who act as if they were better than others, his reaction is anger and retaliation. He wants to hit or slap. He savours revenge, wanting to get back at those who get to him. Does he hit, take revenge? No, he does not. He is fearful of confrontation. He holds on to the anger and hatred as a grudge, even for years. He is waiting for the right moment, maybe when he has a plan for his revenge, probably a devious plan, one in which he cheats or is a hypocrite to get the plan to work. He finds just the right spot to attack and then he will do it, when it is least expected. We know that is how he thinks because he is afraid of sudden attack, and therefore he also will perpetrate them. He must be devious, plotting, and sudden, striking where it will hurt the most, because he feels so small, stupid and picked on by those better than he is.

Finally, there is the issue of dirty and clean. He feels disgusted when dirty. From his perspective, he is meticulous about always being clean. This is far different from the mother's report that he hardly bothers with washing regularly.

He has told us all we need to know. The animal kingdom qualities are very clear: jealous, competition, me versus them, wanting attention and being in the limelight, issues of domination such as being bullied and wanting to dominate, as in his case to be the boss. He does not want to be told what to do, which is the animal feeling of being forced. The kingdom is confirmed by his connection to animals, and the dirty feeling, always needing to be clean.

Choice of remedy
Which grouping within the animal kingdom is he? He hates insects and spiders; they are a symbol for his feelings of hatred, and disgust to such an extent that they make his skin crawl with the very thought of them.

Feeling small, fearful of sudden attack, planning revenge and retaliation but fearful of enacting it are all key features of the arachnid family – spiders. It is also interesting to note that he dreams of and is scared of large cats like the mountain lion. Spiders, in general, have a connection to cats. Cats symbolise everything the spider is not; large, powerful, predator, king of the jungle, sneaky, pounce, graceful and feared. The mountain lion suddenly pounces on him, just as he will spring his well-planned revenge suddenly on those who offend him.

Which spider in particular best fits his life? The symbol that embodies his fearfulness is the heart attack. It is at once sudden and deadly. The spider most known for this symptom is Latrodectus mactans, which is what I prescribed in 200c.

Follow up – one month
Pt: I am much calmer. I do not getting irritated as easily as before. I have more energy. I used to be tired all day. The allergies are much less, with far less runny nose. My acne is much less. I feel stronger when I lift weights. Before I would get irritated at small things, now I can take it better. Things don't bother me as much. In pressure situations, I am much more relaxed. I wake up easily in the morning now. Before I used to be dragging in the morning. I am still bothered by spiders and insects but less. I used to have to wear shoes all the time because I was afraid I would step on them. I still want all my clothes clean.

My headaches are better. I only have them occasionally but they go away in 10 minutes. I used to have to sleep overnight to make them go away. I feel more friendly now. I used to avoid meeting people. I did not like them.

In a dream, I was playing soccer and was repeatedly getting hit with the ball. It seemed as if the ball was coming to me in slow motion and then it would hit me. I couldn't move. I was terrified, frozen with fear.

There was one person I was mad at for a long time then suddenly it just stopped one day. I wouldn't talk to him, then suddenly I did. I gave him another chance. Before I would get really mad, wanting to choke him. I would feel it for days. Now that feeling goes away in a few hours. I am not jealous of anyone anymore.

Follow up summary
I have continued to treat this patient for eight years. During that time he has shown remarkable improvement in every area. His physical

complaints have resolved. He never gets headaches anymore. Occasionally he has some allergic rhinitis return when he is in need of another dose of remedy. His mood has also shown much improvement. He is more confident, less angry and gets along with people far better. When he requires another dose of Lat mac, he will get irritable and feel more jealousy. Otherwise, he does not feel that way.

Further comments on the source
As is often the case, the name of this creature is very telling about its nature. Latrodectus comes from Greek. Latro is a figure in Greek mythology who was robbed of his memory. Dectus is one who bites. Put together, the two are generally translated as 'biting in secret' or 'robber-biter'. Moving from Greece to Rome, the Latin 'mactans' means killing or deadly. All together, the name means 'secret deadly bite' or 'murderous biting robber'. How apt! The quick, deadly pounce from an unobserved source; secretly premeditated, planned and plotted, when you least expect it, sudden death.

A heart attack, more than any other ailment, epitomises this situation of sudden death. We all have seen movies or heard stories of someone seeming perfectly well and the next split second they are on the ground dead – having suffered the ravages of a heart attack. No warning; no defence. Logically a 14-year-old need not be worried about having a heart attack. If his remedy is Latrodectus mactans, he will be.

The suddenness carries with it the implication of preparations, laying in wait, stalking, a devious trap; qualities will known for the arachnoids. Being deceptive, sly, cunning, deceitful, sneaky, devious, threatening, abusive and violent are all part of Lactrodectus mactans. The need to retaliate violently for even the slightest insult, imaged or real, is characteristic.

Other symptoms of Lactrodectus seen in this case are the tendency to be hostile and violent towards the family. The extreme of which is the well-known characteristic of the female black widow spider to devour her mate. In this case, the patient specifically mentions wanting to be aggressive and hit or cut down his brother. For a character who feels small, stupid, bullied and is fearful of confrontation, threatening and beating up on his family members may be the easiest outlet for his pent up rage, hatred and fears.

The three cases of this chapter demonstrate three different ways patients will exhibit their source; naming the source, dreaming of the source and living out its lifestyle. Common to all is the use of source words as the key to joining the patient in his inner world of experience. Every patient has an inner story, an unfamiliar energy causing his non-self behaviour, thoughts, dreams and symptoms. Each patient reveals this energy, the source, to us. It is an exciting and fascinating process to perceive it.

References

1 Korzybski A. A. Non-Aristotelian System and its Necessity for Rigour in Mathematics and Physics, a paper presented before the American Mathematical Society at a, meeting of the American Society for the Advancement of Science in New Orleans LA on December 28, 1931. Reprinted in Science and Sanity, 1933; (S3): 747–61.
2 Dethlesen T., Dahlke R. The Healing Power of Illness Boston: Element Books Ltd, 1990.

7

MOTHER AND CHILD

For decades, it has been standard homeopathic practice in child cases to enquire about the mother and the pregnancy to ascertain if there had been any traumatic events or peculiar symptoms that may have had an impact on the child. Though information was gathered, often it was not quite clear what significance it had or how it may be used to choose a remedy.

The close association, actually an intermingling, of the child and the mother during pregnancy has a profound impact on the state of both. Source-based prescribing utilises information from the mother about her nature, what happened during pregnancy, including any changes, outstanding incidents, traumas, emotionally charged events or distinctive situations. The mother's energy state affects the growing child, even to the point of imprinting her state on the child. Conversely, the child's state may have transmitted to the mother, which is seen as the temporary and out of character symptoms, dreams or desires in the mother during pregnancy. If the mother exhibits new, unusual or distinctively different characteristics during pregnancy, they are important clues to the child's state. The explanation for the stereotypical comment about a pregnant woman suddenly craving pickles, may well be that the foetus wants them!

If, however, the mother's state has not changed during pregnancy, there still can be a link between her state and the infant. It is not the case that all children take on the energy state of their mother. The mother's state as exhibited during pregnancy can be the same as the child if there is a definite link between the symptoms of the child and some aspect of the mother's symptoms. The cases below will demonstrate this very important point.

I do not mean to give fathers short shrift. Both parents are important, each in their own way. The recent trend of more involvement by fathers in the raising of their children is all to the good. Either the mother's state and or the father's state can be present in the child. It can be useful to ask parents which of them the child resembles and in what ways. To use symptoms from a parent's state for the child, there must be a definitive link between the parent and the child through his symptoms or sensations.

Though fathers are now more on the scene, the fact remains that no matter how involved a father is, there is still a special bond between mother and child by the simple biologic fact that mothers bear children and nurse them after birth. A woman's physical structure, hormonal, physiologic and psychological mechanisms are designed for it. The child greatly benefits from this close maternal association. When the mother is in a state of health, it is even more true. Conversely, if the mother is not healthy or experiences a trauma or shocking event, the child can be affected. These play a role as to what state the infant will be in and what remedy he requires. The following cases will elucidate these ideas, showing how to put them to practical use.

Case 7.1   The pregnancy reveals the source

The following case presented by Dr. Sunil Anand and reproduced here with kind permission, demonstrates how the mother's state during pregnancy is linked to the state of the infant, and consequently, his correct remedy. The comments and observations during the consultation are those of Dr. Anand.

Patient
The child is an 18-month-old boy with reflux and coeliac disease who was born one month prematurely. He is still very tiny, but quite active. The clothes he wears would fit a younger child of eight to nine months of age. He has wrinkles behind both his ears. His head is flat from the back on one side. It was a difficult pregnancy because the foetus was not fully developing its lungs. The details are explored later in the case at the appropriate point. As expected with a child of this age, the mother reports the entire case. The child comes into the room wearing a jacket.

Consultation
The case begins spontaneously when I ask his mother to remove it.
M: He gets frequent colds. He gets reflux, so he does not want to eat.
Dr: Tell me the symptoms of his reflux.
M: He burps some liquid or food if we lower the Ranitidine.

Comment Ranitidine is a prescription medication for the treatment of gastric reflux. I observe that the child moves all over the place. He did not want to be held in one place. He was also moving around the table in circles.

Dr: Can you demonstrate how he burps?

Comment The mother demonstrates how the child burps. I find it very useful to see a demonstration of a pre-verbal child's actions and mannerisms. Often simple observation during the case is enough to see what the child does, but if not, the parent should demonstrate it.

M: He coughs out his food or burps or gets hiccoughs after eating. Due to this he has less interest in foods. He eats and drinks very small quantities. This does not allow him to gain weight. He is also very gassy.

Dr: What are the manifestations of that?

M: It is mostly upwards. Occasionally, there is smelly flatus. His stools are generally very strong smelling. It smells of rotten turnips and sometimes has a fishy odour. He gets reflux with most solids so he prefers liquids over solid foods.

Observation He was eating crisps (chips).

M: The anti-emetic helps him to retain things. Even so, due to this he was not gaining weight. He could not digest so many foods so he was tested for coeliac disease. Even though the test was negative, the paediatrician feels that because enzyme responsible for digesting gluten is almost absent and clinical symptoms, he does have indications of coeliac disease. He told us we should avoid wheat as far as possible. He has cautioned us on lactose too.

Dr: Any particular symptoms when he cuts a new tooth?

M: He gets very bad bright red diaper rash as if his bottom was scalded. It almost forms a blister. He gets more than one tooth at a time. There is more drooling with red cheeks. He gets very crabby then and wants to be held and comforted.

Comment Symptoms not related to the chief complaint are as important as information from the presenting complaint itself.

Dr: How does he want to be held and comforted?

Observation The mother demonstrates.

M: He wants to be held still like this –

Comment The mother holds the child in a position similar to a Cina position. Facing the mother, he is lifted up onto and over her shoulder. The mother can rub the back and she demonstrated doing just that.

M: He wants his back to be rubbed. His appetite gets even less than normal when his gums are very sore. Yet, he is averse to soft foods so it is very difficult to get him to eat. He has a lot of temper tantrums and has a very short attention span. At that time, if he cannot get a toy to work, he throws himself on the floor.

Observation Child climbs on table.

Dr: He seems to like climbing?
M: Yes. He loves to climb and look out the window. The child gets a rice cracker from the back of his stroller. He knows it was there. He is very observant and has a good memory.

Observation Child climbs up again.

Dr: He has no fears of falling?
M: No. That is a problem. We have to be around him all the time.
Dr: Is he prone to any other problems?
M: No.
Dr: Say more about him.
M: He loves to dance to music. He goes to the music box and chooses the music he wants and then dances in circles. He uses sign language and points to the music box when he wants the music. We taught him sign language after attending baby sign language class for our older child.

Observation The child demonstrates how he uses sign language. This follows a pattern too: whenever the child hears us saying something he does an imitation of it.

Dr: How does he get along with his sister?
M: Fairly well.

Observation The child dances in circles. This is a distinctive movement and worth taking note of.

Dr: He seems to go around in circles a lot?
M: Not really. Maybe only while he is dancing.
Dr: What else is striking about him?
M: He has such a lovely energy. He is always smiling and affectionate. He loves to be hugged and play and interact with others who come home.

Observation Child goes around in circles on the table while seated. He not only goes in circles while dancing, he is also moving in circles while seated. This is spontaneous and peculiar movement is an important part of the case.

Dr: How much does he sweat?

M: His hands and feet get clammy.

Dr: Any fears?

M: Not yet.

Dr: How was the pregnancy?

M: The alpha beta proteins were very elevated. They suspected some congenital abnormality like spina-bifida. They monitored him very closely. The sonography did not show any abnormality but he was very small. There was a lot of genetic testing and amniocentesis was done once. All was clear. He continued to be very small. They discovered that there was low uterine artery blood flow due to notching. The blood vessels were being compressed by his weight, not allowing blood and nutrients to reach him, hence the low weight gain. Then they monitored him even more carefully. At 30 weeks, they gave me a steroid injection to help his lungs to develop. There was also a risk of me going into eclampsia due to my high blood pressure. At 37 weeks they gave me Natrium Sulphate to avoid seizures. A C-section was advised but I decided to keep going. Finally he was born naturally. His birth weight was only 1840 gms. He was very tiny. He was put under neonatal care so that his body temperature could be maintained. On the day that we were to leave the hospital, they tested him on the car seat with his clothes on. He was ok but then suddenly the oxygen saturation test began to fall very rapidly. At the last minute he stopped breathing. He was taken back to the special care unit once more. His oxygen levels kept fluctuating.

Dr: What were his symptoms when the oxygen levels would fall?

M: He would get very lethargic and tired and his lips would go blue. When he came home, he was very colicky for the first few weeks and would cry a lot. He had very loose stools for the first one month.

Observation Child touches his head to the table.

Dr: Does he do that a lot?

M: Yes. He likes to place his head on cold surfaces. He likes to climb inside things. He goes into the cupboard, climbs into a big empty basket, a toy box or even into an upturned stool space. He loves the water and during bathing loves the water on his head. He puts his face into the water and ends up drinking the bathing water too.

Dr: Any other information about him?

M: He loves being outside, going for little walks and going down the slide.

Dr: Can you say more about the pregnancy?

M: At 32 weeks I could not sleep. I would get into a panic at night.

Dr: Can you describe that sensation of panic?

M: I just needed to be outside. I could not stay indoors. I needed fresh air. I also would get very upset when it would get dark. I just dreaded going to sleep.

Dr: Why?

M: I could not call anyone on the phone at that time. In spite of the cold, I would keep the mattress outside and sleep there. There was a very anxious feeling in my chest inside the house.

Dr: Describe that sensation a bit more and use your hands if you have to.

M: I felt very tight (gestures with hands). It was a feeling of not getting enough oxygen.

Comment Her gesture was like a constriction and compression with all of her fingers together. Later we will see her doodle expresses the same image.

Dr: Say more on that tight sensation and hand gesture.

M: It was like a lump in my chest. I had to breathe in more quickly as if I had to get in more air or oxygen. I had to go outside the house.

Dr: Describe that sensation a bit more and use your hands if you have to.

M: I felt very tight (same gestures with hands). It was a feeling of not getting enough oxygen.

Dr: Can you describe the sensation of wanting more air in its entire sequence from beginning to end?

Comment This is a very important juncture of the case, we are at the point of the vital sensation, the source. She is expressing a feeling with words, gesture and as a symptom that links to the child's symptoms. For these reasons, I ask her to give as much detail as possible by reciting the entire sequence of events and sensations. Speaking form this level, every word will be important and revealing. Her entire being is expressing her inner state. Once at that point, it will be beneficial to ask for a drawing or doodle very soon.

M: I would start getting very restless. I could not be still in one place. I had to be walking around. Then there would be a need for more fresh air. This would make me clench my fists with anxiety.

Dr: What else would you do?

M: Sometimes I would rock a little bit, but going outdoors was better. I did not get very good sleep.

Dr: Say more about your emotional state.

M: I would worry if he were growing inside. All this would get more irrational at night time. I would get a very, very dry mouth with the effort of breathing. Drinking natural spring water from a health food store would help a bit.

Observation   The child attempts to go out by knocking on the door.

M: I could not swallow. It was as if the swallowing reflex would get stuck.
Dr: Can you do a doodle to depict that sensation some more?

Comment   Doodle is the drawing of something clamping tightly, resembling the squeezing of a wind pipe. This is very similar to what she gestured with her hands a few moments ago.

Dr: Talk about the sensation and experience of this doodle?
M: It is like a lump sensation. There is no air. It makes me look up. I just want to stretch and breathe so that I can get in more air. (She demonstrates.)
Dr: Say more.
M: Maybe felt confined. This would get exacerbated at night.
Dr: Look at the doodle and say more.
M: It was a feeling of claustrophobia (she gestures). Things were too small. The room was too small.
Dr: Describe this hand gesture?
M: As if the walls were too close. Then I would feel I need more space. I would want to get out of my small house. Our house is small but at that moment, it would appear even smaller.
Dr: Go back to the labour process and say some more?
M: It had to be induced as there was very slow dilation. I was very tired due to lack of sleep. With every contraction I would throw up but it was more of empty retching as there was not much food in. I was also very constipated during labour. They had to give me an enema as I was very uneasy.
Dr: Say more on that uneasiness?
M: I felt very blocked and hard. The contractions would be even more painful due to the faeces being blocked in. The contractions were very sharp and like a cramp.
Dr: Say more about that sharp cramp?
M: It was almost like a sharp knife with some squeezing. After the enema I felt better.

Observation Child goes around in circles on the carpet. Then he goes in and out of his stroller. The circles continue.

Dr: What else about him?
M: In the hospital they noticed his hypospadias. Also his head shape is flat on one side. He has a blocked tear duct due to which that eye waters and the same eye is smaller than the other.
Dr: At home how does he prefer to be dressed.
M: He wants his socks off.

Comment At this point, I wanted to see how comfortable the child would be if he was unable to see his mother. So I requested the mother to discretely move out of the room without the child being aware of it. Instantly, the child goes hunting for his mother. This need and close attachment to one another, further confirmed the child's remedy. The mother returns with the child.

Dr: What are his cravings in food?
M: He does not like anything that is soft textured. He loves meat and fish. He is averse to sweets.
Dr: What were your cravings during the pregnancy?
M: I craved tomatoes but would throw up with the smell of meat cooking. More than cravings I was averse to fatty and creamy foods and any form of protein.
Dr: What were your dreams?
M: That he is born naturally. He just comes out without any pushing or pain. There was a bright, golden light like a halo around his head.

Comment The above dream is the opposite of what she experienced during labour.

M: In reality, I was 6 cm dilated and I heard the doctors talking that his heart rate was dropping. I was so tired but when I heard that I was suddenly ready to push. I pushed so hard that I got a tear. His was an intrauterine insemination procedure. The donor was from a clinic and unknown to us. My partner is a woman.
Dr: At what point did you feel the need for a child?
M: I always knew that I would have a baby. I wanted one so badly. I am fascinated by the experience of nurturing another human being. The entire process of pregnancy is incredible and amazing for me. It's a miracle and a wonder. I might do it again.

Dr: What is he doing now?
M: He is blowing bubbles. He also pinches and sometimes he bites.

Comment The moment the child heard that, he bit the mother on her shoulder very hard. He is still being held over her shoulder, which give him the right position to easily bite her. This again confirms what we observed earlier – the child tends to replicate what he hears or sees. This observation is significant, as will become clear later. The case-taking is finished now and I am confident of my prescription.

Comments on Dr. Anand's Case Taking

Before Dr. Anand continues with his case analysis, there are some interesting case-taking points to be noted. Dr. Anand follows the child's lead in responding to what movements the child makes. He notes what is distinctive and asks the mother to elaborate about what the child is doing, only for clarification. It is significant that Dr. Anand does *not* ask the mother 'why' the child is moving, thereby avoiding being distracted by the mother's speculation or theories. He takes the movement as a direct communication from the child.

Dr. Anand asks about teething to gather additional clues to the case. Observe that Dr. Anand has gathered information about the child, the chief complaint and noted peculiar movements before asking the mother about the pregnancy. This discussion leads back to the child's symptoms after birth. Notice how Dr. Anand follows the mother's conversation, asking again about the child. Only later does he again pick up the thread and return to the pregnancy. This time a link becomes evident. The child had low oxygen after birth and now the mother relates that she had the sensation of not getting enough air. This vital link between a physical symptom of the child and the mother's sensation during pregnancy is a most important aspect of the case. This tells us that the mother's state in pregnancy will reveal the remedy the child needs. We can fully explore this sensation.

The spontaneous hand gesture accompanying the mother's description is further emphasis that Dr. Anand is on the right track and close to the source. Now his questioning is focused completely in this area, asking the exact details of that experience from start to finish. Any detail about this sensation will be fruitful. The mother stays in that state, reliving it more and more. Her entire being is expressing her inner state. Once at that point, it will be beneficial to ask for a drawing or doodle, the non-verbal rendition of her state. The words that come up now are those connected to the source.

Dr. Anand asks about the labour process at a well-chosen point in the case. From all the information collected so far, he is now aware that the remedy is in the second row of the periodic table. He will explain how he came to that conclusion himself in the case analysis below. For now, we are examining the method of case-taking to understand the process. This question asked this moment is serving to clarify and confirm which remedy in that group. From this point on, all other questions are confirmatory.

Analysis – Dr. Sunil Anand's comments
The child's problem list and characteristics include reflux, offensive stools with a rotten turnip or fish odour, failure to thrive, early caries of his teeth, gluten and lactose intolerance, recurrent colds, hypospadias and a blocked tear duct. During the consultation other useful characteristics came out. There is a very strong bond between the mother and child. They even seem to be incomplete without each other. He wants attention, especially her attention. He gets physical with mother, wanting to be held closely, but also even biting her. He likes to imitate, repeating a structured pattern. He was hyperactive and could not be contained. He was always moving, climbing and moving in circles. On the other hand he likes being contained when he is held closely or when he is in his stroller. He closes the roof of it to make a smaller space. He has no fear of heights and likes cold surfaces and loves water.

The mineral kingdom features are that he desires a support system and familiarity in the form of being so attached to his mother. There is a very strong bond. He follows sequences, replicates and imitates. The indications for row two minerals are even more pronounced and help to confirm the choice of this kingdom. As was mentioned in my previous case of Adamas, the primary theme of row two is separation; fear of separation from your source. There is no evidence of identity issues that would take us to row three. With breathing problems, asphyxiation and the strong urge for air, we are still at the survival level inherent in row two. There is a labour crisis and the child needs air. Love of water also points to row two, as a reminder of the amniotic fluid and the mother's womb.

Distinctive and peculiar is that the child has no fears, which are usual and strong in row two elements, especially Borax and Nitrogen. In this case there are other source words pointing to a mineral that is in gas form above and beyond the symptoms typical for a lack of air, asphyxia and cyanosis. These include the need for cold air and cold surfaces, cannot be contained, easy collision, light and tiny and the need to escape. The child climbs as often as he can, as a gas rises. In row two we see Oxygen that easily fits all the source words and symptoms of the case.

The source words and themes for Oxygen include air, suddenness, panic, cyanosis, exhaustion, circle, easy exhaustion, sudden crisis, restriction, high energy, restless moving, anaesthesia and strong attachment alternating with the need to be free. The qualities include liking open space, freedom and movement ameliorates. Both the mother and child felt the need for air and wanting to be outside. The child was always moving. The source also is known to have the sensation of being stuck, which the child demonstrated when his swallowing reflex would get stuck. Dehydration and dryness are also characteristics. The mother commented that she felt better drinking natural spring water from the health food store. How easy it would be to overlook that small and seemingly insignificant comment. Yet, it is important. Bottled spring water has a higher oxygen content that regular water. Again we see the source expressing itself, even in what might appear as the most minor of details.

Choice of remedy

Swan carried out a proving with potentised Oxygen. Three symptoms stood out; flatulence, nasal mucous, and cough. Chemically, when the gas is cooled, the particles are moving slowly. It can even be cooled to the point of becoming a liquid or solid. When heated, they can move so fast that liquid oxygen is used for rocket propulsion fuel.

There is another mineral presenting itself too; Carbon. It can be difficult to differentiate because Carbon has many qualities in common with Oxygen such as the need for air and the sensation of things getting smaller or of the room being too small as well as tending to want to get into closed spaces. The most telling symptom is the alternation between dependence and wanting to break away. The child demonstrates this by his wanting to be held closely, but from that position he bites his mother aggressively.

Both the Oxygen and the Carbon and the gaseous qualities must be taken into consideration. I prescribed Carbo oxygenisatum, more familiarly known as carbon monoxide. The remedy was administered as LM 3 once daily for two weeks. The LM potency was chosen on the basis of the past history of acute crises and the child being on medications.

Among the known symptoms of Carbo oxygenisatum are anaesthesia, insensibility and cyanosis and dryness of usually moist internal parts such as the mouth.

Most interesting is that a distinctive characteristic of the child, his propensity to move in a circle, is noted throughout the case. This observation is the fulcrum of the case from the point of observation and the energy of the case. Carbo oxygenisatum is the only remedy in the following rubric:

■ Generalities: inclination to turn in a circle.

Though I used the many new methods to take the case and arrive at the remedy, this case, with this defining rubric, highlight the continued need for intelligent use of the repertory, which sadly is totally ignored by even seasoned practitioners much to their peril. Provings and the repertory are still very significant sources of useful information to guide us and we must continue to refer to them.

Follow up – one month

M: The reflux is better. He says his tummy hurts sometimes; maybe he's hungry. If I give him food, he will eat a little. He doesn't point to his throat now when his tummy hurts. He is not on Pediasure anymore. He is not night waking much anymore. He will cry but we leave him alone and he sleeps.

Dr: How about the circles?

M: Occasionally he does it, just now and again. He used to do it a lot. He puts his head to the floor, is on his knees and pushes himself in a line or in a circle. He gets a rug burn on his forehead. Since the remedy he is sleeping more and saying he's hungry. That is different now. He grew 1 cm this month and has started to gain weight. We noticed that his vocabulary has expanded a lot since his last visit. He looked good, happy and was very engaging. He has captured all our hearts! We feel that the remedy has definitely touched him.

Comment This was also the first time that the child had come in without remnants of a cold. Soon after the LM the mother was able to stop the anti-emetics.

M: His stools became more solid and less smelly. His colds did not recur as much and they subside on their own without any medication. He could tolerate more foods.

We have decided to postpone the surgery for the hypospadias.

Comment Phimosis and other genital related abnormalities are common to carbon remedies. I reduced the frequency of LM to once in four days. The respite in symptoms continued even after weaning of the dose.

Follow up – six months
The response to the LM dose is not as good as earlier. His symptoms still would respond but slowly. By now his vitality was better. He has been gaining weight and height. He has been tolerating other foods better. At this point the LM was discontinued and a single dose of a 200c was given and he immediately responded.

Further comments on the source
Carbo oxygenisatum or carbonous oxide is known for its anaesthetic and toxic properties. Carbon oxygenisatum (carbon monoxide) is one of the main air pollutants and is also highly toxic, causing loss of consciousness, stupor and anaesthesia. Carbonous oxide is one of the few substances that can, like oxygen, combine with, or unite itself to the red corpuscle. Hence its poisonous action depends principally upon the displacement of oxygen, with consequent suffocation. Of course, lack of oxygen in animal tissue invariably leads to a general disturbance, the central phenomena of which appear in respiratory, cardiac symptoms and other symptoms. The picture is one of asphyxia.

The essence of Carbo oxygenisatum has several aspects. On one hand, the security of being in the mother's womb is very comforting but at a certain point there has to be a separation in order to survive. It is important to experience freedom and the ability to survive by taking that first breath. But once out, the child yearns to go back from time to time and seek the comfort of the mother. The feeling of the child is the insecurity of wondering whether he will be able to survive this toxic world in the total absence of a mother or a secure environment. The child seeks the protected and pure environment by being close to the mother figure, to whom he gives affection. As close as he is, he also feels the normal need to separate. He exhibits resistant behaviour, directed mainly at the mother, even to the point of aggression designed to separate.

The aspect of imitation and replication is seen in most carbons, referred to as the 'carbon copy' syndrome. There is a need to climb without any fear of heights. Circular movement. Of course we expect to see the desire for more oxygen. What is interesting is that this desire can prompt a craving for spring water or carbonated drinks, which contain high levels of oxygen!

As the final comment about this case, it should be noted that either parent's state can have a significant link to that of the child. This case demonstrates the significance of the mother's predominant state during pregnancy. What is important is for the link to be correlated without any imposition or prejudice. Only when there is a natural connection is there relevance of the mother's state during pregnancy. We can also place emphasis on the entire labour process and any significance dreams of the mother. The case also highlights the relevance of doodles and observations, especially in pre-verbal children. Both of these helped reach the core of the case and the vital sensation more directly. These can also be used for older children and adults when one is faced with a block or when the case is deeply compensated. These are extremely useful tools in many cases.

Dr. Sunil Anand's case clearly demonstrates the useful and even essential information that is derived from careful, judicious and skilful investigation of the mother's state, before and during pregnancy. Most instructive is the elucidation of how important it is to detect the connection between the mother and the child's state through common feelings, sensations and experiences.

Case 7.2 The dream reveals the source

What do we do when that connection is not evident; when there is no apparent link between the mother's state or symptoms and the child? The first answer is to keep investigating, patiently using all the tools at our disposal such as the inquiry into the dreams, past history, hobbies, doodles, recurrent words, peculiar symptoms or statements. Yet, sometimes even that is not enough to clarify the link we seek. In the event that there is no link found, we have to make certain presumptions about that connection. Naturally, that is not the best circumstance, and only done when necessary. The next short case will demonstrate such a situation. The mother's state is clear but there is only a presumptive link to the child.

Patient
The patient is a three-month-old infant girl, whose whole body is completely covered in weeping, excoriated eczema. With such extensive dermatitis in a non-verbal patient, it is unlikely that I will be able to find any peculiar characteristic on which to begin the case. I am prepared that the mother may hold the key to helping the child. Both the mother and father accompany the child and participate in providing information about their child.

M and F: She has had no immunisations. We don't believe in them. The first we noticed that anything was wrong was what the doctors called cradle cap. She had that rash on the top of her head and a few red marks on her forehead. Then the rash started on the back of her legs and forehead. Then went to the right side of her face. It is red and rough. Then it extended to the front of her arms and front of her legs and thighs. Now it is everywhere. The week before this visit it had really kicked up. She is always scratching and we can't stop her. She scratches until it bleeds and the skin is raw. It is in her ears and all over her scalp.

Consultation
Dr: What is her nature?
M and F: She is a wonderful child. She is easy going and very good natured. She likes attention and wants to be held but we can also put her down without her fussing. She sleeps with us and is calm and quiet, sleeping well at night.

Comment For a child who is so afflicted with an itching rash, she is very calm and good-natured. She is not irritable or fussy. There is no information about the rash other than the usual symptoms expected with such rapidly spreading eczema. Even the fact that the problem first showed up at the bends of the knees is not peculiar enough to be of help. I pursue the investigation by going right to the pregnancy.

Dr: Tell me about the pregnancy.
M: It was fine. I had some morning sickness but not too badly. Towards the end I got irritable because I couldn't move around. I had a caesarean section with general anaesthesia.
Dr: What was going on in your lives during the pregnancy?
M: We were having a lot of stress about finding a place to live. We had moved in with my parents. It was really stressful being there. They put a lot of pressure on us to move out. I really felt that they were rushing us out

of the house. They were very unhappy and disappointed that I was pregnant. It was a very sad time for us because of that. We did not tell my parents for a long time about the pregnancy. If I had my way, I would never have told anyone. My father just thought I was getting fat. When we finally told them, my mother cried a lot. We both wanted to get out of that house as soon as possible but there was nowhere to go.

Dr: Tell more about this.

M: It was terrible growing up. I always feel not accepted. I tended to rebel against my parents. They thought I was troublesome and rebellious. My parents always said I was going to the devil. They sent me away. We were supposed to be on vacation only but they left me here at the school without telling me what was going on. I felt they were giving up on me as if I was a really bad kid. Now that I am back in their house, they make me feel the same. My dad always told me that I was not presentable. My parents never showed me any affection. They never lifted me up as parents usually do with their children. I was unloved by my father. I can never put it into words.

Dr: Tell me more about your nature.

M: I get obsessed with things. I do weird things like check things over and over. I am obsessed about cleanliness. I am loyal and a good friend.

F: She tends to be hard on herself. She does not like to be criticised, yet she criticises herself all the time. She puts herself down.

M: I have low self-esteem. I am not happy with myself. I feel threatened by thin women. I am extremely jealous of the thinner women. When I think about them, I feel rage and anger. It is an uncontrollable rage. I get so angry at myself because I don't lose weight. I just seem to gain weight and get bigger and bigger. I am convinced that my husband will leave me for a thinner woman. This happens when I am around my thinner friends. I am jealous and envious to have a better body. Maybe it is because my father always made bad comments about my body. He told me I was disgusting to look at. He still does it to this day. He will say, 'Who is prettier and who is fatter?' I have rage against my body and rage against skinny girls.

Observation She has a slight lisp while talking, more noticeable when she talks about skinny girls or her rage.

Dr: Tell me more.

M: It was felt so hurtful and painful. I would lock myself in my room. I always feel better talking to my girlfriends. With them, I was outgoing.

Dr: Tell me more about your nature.

M: I get really angry when my husband doesn't keep things clean. I am anxious about who is in the room with me. I am very embarrassed about my appearance. I know I should be thin and not gain weight. Then I am embarrassed about comments made in front of others. I feel worse when they look at me. Why are they always looking at me? I know it is because I am so big. I feel such anger and rage that I end up leaving and weeping all day by myself. I want to run away and hide forever.

Dr: What dreams do you have?

M: I have dreams of flying. I feel great and I am in control of my life. One terrible dream was that I had ants crawling all over me. It was disgusting and I felt all creepy, crawly and itching. I want them off of me. The other dream is very embarrassing to tell you. I had it a very long time ago.

Dr: Say only what you feel comfortable saying.

M: I should tell you. I had a dream that I was with a bunch of girls in gym class who were friends of mine. We all dropped our underwear and our private places were exposed. My private part grew very large and long like a man's. It was extremely embarrassing. I think it is more embarrassing telling it to you.

Comment Despite how long ago the dream occurred, she remembers the details of it. Another feature is the strong emotional reaction the dream creates, then and now. Both of these factors make the dream important.

M: I had fearful dreams when I was pregnant and after she was born. I dreamt that I left her in the car seat and in the bath. I leave for a second and when I come back, she is under water and not breathing.

Dr: What was the feeling in those dreams?

M: I felt panicked and terrified. I had done wrong again and killed my child. I am so awful. I do not like those dreams. They made me scared.

Dr: Each of you tell me more about your natures.

F: I have a strong sense of right and wrong. I will stand up strongly for a principle. I think I am intelligent and hard working. I certainly have high expectations of myself. I don't mind saying exactly what is on my mind. I am not shy. I was shy when I was younger because I had a stammer. I had speech therapy that helped and it is gone now.

M: As I said, I rebelled against my parents. One way was to like heavy rock music. I was happy that my parents hated my music. Since age 12, I wrote weird poems and about sex, even though I did not have sex until age 16.

Overall, I was just sad and lonely, being in love with the idea of being in love with someone. It really started after my parents left me at that school. How could they do this to me. How could any parent just abandon their child? I was all alone. I wrote in my diaries constantly. Mostly I wrote about boys I liked. I have been doing that since I was six years old.

Dr: Any fears?

M: I am really afraid of dogs, I am sure they will attack me. I know it is silly but I think they will.

Dr: Anything else you would like to add?

F: We forgot to mention that she (the mother) was vaccinated during pregnancy and had rubella vaccine the day after birth. We are against them, but the doctors scared her and they did it anyway.

Analysis

The child cannot speak for herself other than through her symptoms. Unfortunately, her symptoms are all general, common, none of them having the distinctive or peculiar features that are helpful. Focusing on the mother, I will look for connections and links between the mother and the child.

The mother's nature has many animal features. She is jealous, envious, feels put down and is overly concerned with her appearance. There is a strong sexual element to her personality from a young age. Although not overly sexual in her actions, her thoughts and writings have been pre-occupied with sexuality. These are characteristics of the animal kingdom. There are also indications for a snake remedy. She feels persecuted, looked at and despised. Dreams of flying also point to snakes, (among other animals). Lisping is also a snake trait. Her lisp was noticeable especially when she talked about those topics that were aggravating to her. She also did not have many symptoms that would have confirmed a snake remedy. She was not loquacious, had no fear or dreams of snakes, did not have heat flushes, choking sensations, desire retaliation or exhibit overt aggressiveness. Despite the absence of these typical snake features, there is enough in her case to pursue the snake family.

Choice of remedy

Now it is time to consider what is peculiar in the case. The embarrassing dream holds the most unusual finding. As mentioned, the intensity of her feeling, the details remembered after so many years, highlight the dream for consideration. In the dream her body part enlarges. She has that same feeling in her daily life about her body as a whole. She feels that she gets bigger and bigger. Just like in the dream, her body enlarging makes her embarrassed. This connection between her physical condition and the dream further emphasises the dream's importance. What snake is particularly known for enlargement? Of course, all snakes have an overall sensation of constriction and enlargement, but for which is it an overriding sensation? Only Cenchris is listed in the repertory for the peculiar sensation and delusion of specific body parts being enlarged. Additionally the whole body feels enlarged to the point of bursting. Is it too far afield to say that her large body makes her burst into tears? She doesn't burst any other way: she doesn't scream, hit or throw things; just tears.

Can I confirm this choice? Kent's 1888 proving of Cenchris reveals the symptom, 'Itching all over the body, flying all over the body.' Here is our first hint of a connection to the child. Recall the mother's other dream of ants crawling all over her body making her itch. Hering's proving of Lachesis in 1828 and 1834 produced the following: 'Violent itching on the scalp, as from ants. Violent itching on the scalp, and over the whole body.' In the absence of other common symptoms and connections, this one is enough for me. I prescribe Cenchris 30 to the child.

Follow up – one month
M and F: Immediately after the dose, she fell asleep and slept for 5 hours in a row for the first time. Her left side started clearing up right away. Overall there is much less discharge from the rash. Her legs and arms are greatly improved. She is not yet 100% better, or all the way cured but she is so much better. She still has some scabs from scratching but they heal very quickly. Her cradle cap is all gone and she has much less scratching. We noticed that she is losing her hair in patches. She wants to be held and carried all the time. We can't put her down as before. She wants attention all the time.

Follow up – two months
M and F: Her torso is completely clear, as well as her limbs. Overall the rash is much improved. We are happy that she now can sit longer by herself with less need to be carried.

Follow up – three months
M and F: She is laughing more. She smiles! We did not realise that was absent until she started smiling and laughing recently. She is so happy. We can leave her longer by herself without holding her. Her cheeks and face are completely clear and her hair is growing back in places.

Follow up – five months
M and F: Her head is completely smooth and without any rash. She is more interested in the world around her. She always smiles and laughs and engages.

Follow up – nine months
M and F: Overall skin is much improved. There is hardly any rash left. There is only some slight rash on the back of her head and the back of legs. That is where it all started.
    She sleeps through the night.

Follow up – one year
M and F: All her skin is perfectly clear. It is rare to see her scratch. All her hair has returned.

Summary of follow ups
I have continued to treat this child. She has done extremely well with Cenchris, staying on that remedy for four years. At that point she had not had any rash for years. As she grew, other characteristics appeared. She was an intensely shy child, being unable to release her parents' hand or move from their lap. She buried her head in their shoulder or chest rather than be looked at. She had large neck lymph nodes especially when she had a cold. She also developed a stammer, made worse when she was looked at. Recall that her father also had a stammer as a youth. For this and other reasons, her remedy was now changed to Baryta carb. She has remained on that remedy successfully for the last eight years. She is now a lively, social, pleasant and charming 12-year-old.

Case 7.3   The mother reveals the source

Here is another case from Dr. Sunil Anand. It demonstrates how the mother's general state is linked to the child and how the child enacts it. The comments and observation during the consultation are those are those of Dr. Anand.

Patient
Nineteen month old infant boy with recurrent upper respiratory infections with otitis media.

Right away, I observe that the child is unusually shy, so I spend some time initially building trust and comfort for the child.

Consultation
Dr: Tell me about the child.
M: He is a happy, easy-going kid. He is learning new words. He loves putting his hand in the fish bowl. He does not scream, he only whines a bit. He plays games with me. For example, he crawls and expects me to crawl and catch him and then we wrestle. He gives me hundreds of kisses but he does not like being smooched on the lips. He does drool. He has to be very careful getting off his cycle.
Dr: Tell more about his personality.
M: Daycare attendants say he is not a physical boy. I see that he loves playing in the water during his bath.
Dr: So water figures a lot with him; the bath and his hand in the fish bowl?
M: Yes, but he does not like his hair to be washed or cut.
Dr: Say more about this.
M: He has high energy. He plays with his hair a lot.

Observation She gestures quite spontaneously and starts gently rubbing several fingers together, one against the other, rolling her hair between them. As she does this, I see her visibly relax; her face softens and eyes look upwards as she enters a zone of comfort and peace, almost ecstasy.

Dr: In what way?
M: It's comforting for him. He plays with the top of his hair a lot.
Dr: Say more about this.
M: He plays with my hair too. There is a woman at the daycare with curly hair. He does not know what to do with it! I do that a lot with my hair too. I like the smooth, silky feel. He likes the smooth, silky feel. Whenever I get him back from the daycare he holds my hand with his free hand.

Dr: Apart from hair, is there anything else of the same kind of texture that he likes to feel?
M: He likes the cat, stuffed toys and finger puppets
Dr: Tell me about your habit.
M: I have also found touching my hair very comforting.
Dr: When do you do this?
M: When I am tired I do it. I have done it ever since I was a kid.
Dr: What is the sensation when you do that?
M: Smooth and soft. I like it when it is wet and cold to touch, like now.

Observation The mother demonstrates.

Dr: Tell more about that sensation.
M: It is like putting your hand in a shallow stream with moss in it, as the water passes through the fingers.
Dr: Tell about the feeling of the moss or the water.
M: The feeling of the moss and the water is that the moss does not pass through your fingers.
Dr: Describe the moss sensation.
M: Soft, slimy and cold.
Dr: Say more on soft, slimy and cold.
M: It is like an ice cube but not that harsh.

Comment Here is a block. She does not go deeper. This is the right time to ask for a doodle.

Dr: Can you do a doodle while you experience this sensation?

Observation Doodle 1: At first she draws a plant with the first leaves going upwards and deep roots beneath. She ponders what she has drawn and it does not seem complete to her. Then she draws waves of water on the leaves giving the impression of the leaves being partially submerged in a running river stream.

Dr: Talk about this.
M: It is a plant that is under water. It is soft, like when it flows back and forth and there is high energy.

Observation Again she gestures. Her hands are slowly and gently fanning sideways back and forth as she demonstrates the sensation of a plant under water and the water is flowing over it, waving back and forth. Her face is still relaxed and calm, expressing a very comfortable feeling.

Dr: Do the action of back and forth.

Observation She demonstrates the back and forth movement again.

Dr: Talk of this gesture and sensation.
M: It is a plant in a stream of water. It is rooted but the water makes it go back and forth.
Dr: How strong is it rooted?
M: Not incredibly strong but strong enough that the water cannot pull it. If you pulled at it, it would come out easily. It is that kind of a root system.
Dr: Say more about its root system.
M: It is anchored in something that is soft like a clay bed or the bottom of a riverbed. It is sort of bushy. I imagine something like clay where it can have roots that are deep enough.

Observation She gestures with her fingers pointing downwards showing that the plant roots are embedded within the soft ground.

Dr: Describe your relationship with your child.
M: We are well connected. After two guesses, I know why he is upset. There is ebb and flow. There are his needs and my response to them.

Observation She gestures again in response to ebb and flow, which is quite similar to the gesture she made showing the back and forth.

Dr: Say more on ebb and flow and this gesture.
M: It is like a conversation without words. It is like our souls are talking to each other.

Comment Ebb and flow comes up in both the discussion and the doodle, so I will investigate here more.

Dr: Visualise ebb and flow and say more. Can you do a doodle again while experiencing this sensation?

Observation Doodle 2: She draws a person sitting on a rocking chair but the motion is to rock sideways. There is a semi-circle indicating moving sideways.

M: It is like when you sit on a rocking chair, a sideways rocking chair as I am doing it. I feel like I am moving sideways.

Observation She rocks sideways with a fan-like movement. The movement is similar to the back and forth and the ebb and flow gestures. The motions are all similar despite using different words.

Comment This is an interesting, peculiar sensation, which I will explore.

Dr: Say more about what you are experiencing.
M: It is comforting, relaxing and reminds me of sleeping.
Dr: In what way?
M: It's a nice way to go to sleep, like lying on a hammock. It is warm and comforting. You are warm in your core.
Dr: Say more.
M: It radiates from the core. Radiates out, like the sun. It is like when you put paint inside a glass of water and the way it disperses.
Dr: Did you feel the same sensation of being well connected even when he was in the womb?
M: No. I felt exactly the opposite.
Dr: Talk about the opposite.

Comment The sensation and its opposite are two sides of the same coin. Often while probing its opposite, the inner sensation is derived more easily.

M: My husband left me when I was five months pregnant. There was a total disconnect. I did not want to be in my own skin anymore. Even when he was born, I did not look at him. He was going to complicate my life. I felt trapped. You feel kind of trapped with maximum energy.

Observation She gestures by moving both hands up to her upper chest and lower throat area. The hands come together but are not clenching.

Dr: Talk about that sensation.
M: Like you are just suffocating.
Dr: Talk about trapped and suffocated.
M: Its like you are underneath water and you can't get to the top. There is a sensation of everything being closed and tight. There was a total disconnect from my child. That is how I felt then. Now I like him a lot. It was as if you are stuck in a small, confined space.

Comment When the words 'as if' are used to describe a sensation, the patient is very close to the vital sensation. I often use it as a form of a question if there is difficulty on the part of the patient in elaborating their inner sensation. For example, I will ask the patient, 'You feel as if what?'

M: I felt stuck, confined and suffocated like being in a pipe, like having a straitjacket on.
Dr: Tell about a straitjacket.
M: Your arms are like this. You can't move them. Your rib cage can't expand and you can't take a good breath. You have to take little breaths to survive. It is like a black cloud.

Observation She pulls her arms in close to her body, as close as possible, being pulled in closer than when she talked of being trapped. She is showing that she can't breathe.

Dr: Can you say how you felt when your husband left you?
M: I was desperately upset.

Comment The miasm is getting confirmed, since the remedy should be close to one that feels desperate.

M: Two weeks before I had him, there was a tremendous, paralysing fear. It was like a black cloud that follows you everywhere.
Dr: Tell me about the black cloud.
M: It was dark and cold. It is like you have dug a really black hole in your backyard. It is cold down there. It was a feeling of heaviness. There was a trapped and suffocated sensation. Yet, I just did not want to get out of it. I had no energy. I was so low. I did not have the energy to even try to get out. Earlier I wanted to get out. At this point, I had no more energy left.

Comment Once again, the Tubercular miasm is being confirmed. The desperation indicated a miasm close to the Cancer miasm earlier.

M: I had paralysing fear. I recall not being able to function well. I was weeping, but could not think. I would lie to people because I did not want to go out or meet anyone. I just wanted to be alone by myself. I felt desperate. I had imagined how my life would be with a partner and I did not have that now.

Comment I have a very good picture of the mother's state during the pregnancy and her feeling and sensations. I also have identified the miasm. For more information, I go to the chief complaint. You have to be flexible about the chief complaint, especially in children. Once the vital sensation and link, if any, is established, the chief complaint is understood better. That is why I usually investigate it later in the case, as I am doing now. However, there are times when the emphasis of the case is on the chief complaint from the beginning. Then it can be better to probe that fully and then proceed to confirm the other levels.

Dr: Describe his ear infections.
M: With each cold that he gets, it goes into his ears and there is high fever and he is in pain. He doesn't scream with the pain but he gets irritable. He has to be held and caressed. There is a green nasal discharge and he loses his appetite. His cough wakes him up. He has had six courses of antibiotics in the past six months.
Dr: Tell more about the child.
M: He doesn't like his upper arms to be touched. There was an incident of someone holding him by the arms and picking him up. He howled when that was done. He is very sensitive to his environment. He senses when his father will come home. He stops and stares if he hears a baby crying or people fighting.
Dr: Have you had problems with your periods?
M: No. Except that they came when I was 15.
Dr: Any muscle or joint related issues?
M: No. In fact I play a lot of sport so my physical fitness is very good.
Dr: Any other illness for you that involves pain?
M: I have had irritable bowel syndrome (IBS) for many years.
Dr: Tell me about the IBS and your childhood.
M: It is anxiety and anticipation related. I have the anxiety of not reaching the bathroom in time. Travelling became difficult and being in a car for long was a problem. I would anticipate trouble. Otherwise I was a happy child, well organised and perfect. I was always nice to people. Now that I don't have the energy, I am more selective. I am sensitive. I remember reading a poem about a harpoon striking a whale. I started to cry while relating this poem. It was very embarrassing.
Dr: Tell about any pain and IBS.
M: There is a lot of pain. It is like an intestinal knotting, like a rope with a bunch of knots in it. It gets tighter and it releases. It is like an old rope that prickles in a painful way, like poking your hand on a porcupine. It is a sharp pain that causes me to double over.

Comment The confirmation of the link between the mother and child is seen by the love for water and the feel of soft things. The aversion to being held by the arms in the child links to the strait jacket experience in the mother. Both have acutely sensitive natures. Therefore I am on solid ground in using the mother's symptoms and characteristics to prescribe for the child.

Analysis
The extreme sensitivity of both mother and child is very clear, having been stated outright by the mother. There can be no doubt that the child needs a remedy from the plant kingdom. Additional confirmations come from the plant imagery from the mother's doodle and gestures. She spoke of the root of a plant rather than a tree. Plants are more easily uprooted than trees, as follows her description. The most important indicator for the plant kingdom is their tremendous sensitivity. The other very essential feature of the plant kingdom is the presence of a particular sensation *and its opposite*. It is possible to find sensations in patients who need remedies from any kingdom, however, only the plant kingdom has the pair of polarities – a sensation and its direct opposite.

Choice of remedy
The specific perceived sensation directs us to the particular plant family differentiating it from all others. The sharp pains, and the opposite in the form of the soft and silky sensation of the hair, take me to the Ranunculaceae family. The trapped, desperate and suffocated feelings confirm the Tubercular miasm. I will prescribe the tubercular remedy of the Ranunculaceae family, which is designated by Sankaran to be Cimicifuga racemosa or Black Cohosh.

Confirming symptoms of Cimicifuga racemosa include a powerful, overwhelming feeling of depression as if enveloped in a black cloud. She gives a thorough description of feeling this after her husband left.

In this case, it could be misleading to think of the trapped, straitjacket feeling as the sensation of the case. She displayed a lot of energy and some gestures while speaking of this feeling. Why is this not the sensation pointing to the plant family Euphorbiaceae, for example, with its hidebound, tied, encircled sensations? A very critical point of differentiation is to correctly identify what is the central sensation and what is not. In this case 'soft' and the polarity 'sharp' are the pair of sensations. When she is feeling the softness, she goes to a place of comfort, peace, connection and relaxation. I witnessed her in that state of sublime peace. When she is feeling the sharpness of not being connected, she is completely desperate, all symbolised by the images and feelings of being underwater, trapped and in a straitjacket. This is her reaction to the lack of softness; it is the miasm. In this case, it is the tubercular miasm.

I arrived at Cimicifuga racemosa using the new methods of miasms, sensations and plant families. However, I do not forget our foundation, provings and repertory. Confirming rubrics for the case include the following:

- Mind: Fear of death: saw wires encaging him.
- Mind: Delusions: is caught in wires.
- Mind: Delusions: heavy black clouds enveloped her.
- Skin: Soft feeling.

Cimicifuga racemosa was given in the 200c potency.

Follow up – six weeks
The child got an acute upper respiratory infection. The attack was much milder than the previous ones. The plan was to wait for 48 hours because it was not that bad. The child settled down in two days without the need for another dose. Since then the child continues to be well. He has had no ear infections or high fever.

Additional comments
There are many aspects of Dr. Sunil Anand's case-taking that are worthy of note. Early in the consultation, within the first few questions, the mother connects herself with the child by comparing their exactly similar preferences for a smooth and silky sensation. Of course, a 19-month-old has not told her that he likes smooth and silky. She presumes it because she does and his actions are the same as hers. We can presume he also likes the same sensation. The important thing is that significant similarities between mother and child are revealed so early. This allows us to learn about the child from the mother with confidence because the connection has been demonstrated.

I want to point out the significance of the stage in the interview when Dr. Sunil Anand asks the mother to make a doodle. She had mentioned some source words in connection to a very interesting image. She has gone from touching hair to the smooth and silky texture of the hair to the water and moss. From the reality of her habit, one that she shares with her son, she goes to the imaginary world of the running water flowing over her fingers. That was the turning point of passing from the outside conscious world, to her inner reality. Once there, it is always our aim to stay there because there is where the source is. Anything coming from this place will be useful source information. Dr. Anand gently asks her to say more. She says the same word, soft, but also two new ones, slimy and cold. Then she mentions an ice cube that is harsh. Now we have lost the path.

Why not ask about the new words and the ice cube? How do I know that she is off the path, not at the source anymore? This is a very important question and fundamental to success with source-based prescribing. What is source information and what is not? Some aspects of the answer can be put into words and other times it has to do with the 'feel' or 'energy' of the interaction with the patient.

In this case, there was an ease or flow travelling the path from hair to smooth to water flowing. It was natural, spontaneous and genuine. Once she said slimy and cold, something had shifted and it did not seem as if she was speaking from her experience but from a concept about moss. When she said ice cube, I was certain that she was thinking logically about cold and not connected to the sensation she started with – the smooth silky hair and water. I am attempting to put into words a very subtle change that occurs with patients. Of course, Dr. Anand was aware of the change too, since he stopped the direction he was going and took another route, asking for the doodle, to get her back to the right path to the source.

After the doodle, the patient talks about water, soft and the back and forth flow. This connects to the previous reference to the flowing of the water and softness. She has gotten back on track. If there was any doubt, it is dispelled by the accompanying gestures. She has returned successfully to the source where there is the stream of water, soft and movement. In this context the new word 'root' is significant.

She now goes from 'back and forth' to 'ebb and flow', connected by the same gesture. What is the ebb and flow? It is the relationship she has with her child. The ebb and flow are his needs and her responses to him; energy and communication flowing between them. She describes the experience as if their souls were talking to each other. Starting with the habit they have in common, that of touching her hair, she has travelled a direct route to their two souls talking. For this mother, when her child touches her hair he is touching her soul.

Sense the difference between how she is before and after the doodle by what she says and does. I know it is difficult to do with only what you are now reading, without hearing or seeing her, but it is still possible to perceive the difference. With moss, cold, slimy and ice-cube, she was speaking from her logical, thinking mind. Her discussion was flat, lifeless and theoretical. When you sense that from a patient, you are not at the source.

The source is their truth emanating from their personal experience. There is no reason or rationale: it is pure experience. Logic has no place. When you hear logic and thinking, by definition, you know you are not where you want to be. Once the patient returns to the source, he speaks with an authenticity that is unmistakable. There is life back in the case.

Gestures and other body movements often occur at the level of the source because words do not suffice to express the experience. That is what occurred in this case.

Once you start experiencing the difference between a patient's logical talking as contrasted to his speaking from the source in your own cases, you will be able to easily identify when that change takes place. You will get to the point of knowing when the patient is at the source by the quality of the interaction.

This is not to say that there is no value at all in things said at other times. All information is important. However, all homeopaths must have the skills to know what state the patient was in when they gave the information in order to know what priority to give it and how to utilise it. I will emphasise what I had mentioned in a previous chapter: the homeopath follows the patient's lead but must always know where he is.

Case 7.4 The child *in utero* reveals the source

So far the cases have been examples of the mother's state influencing or revealing the child's. That is not always the situation. It can also happen that the child's state will display itself through the mother as evidenced by her showing symptoms that are a marked departure from her normal state. The following case demonstrates this circumstance.

Patient
The patient is a newborn girl who was born by scheduled caesarean section at 38 weeks without any problems. She weighed 2.5 kg. (5 lb. 7 oz) at birth. She is the second child, having a three-year-old brother. Her mother has been treated since 1996 with Androctonus and her father has

also been treated successfully for four years. Her first evaluation was 11 days after birth because of difficulty breathing and maintaining oxygenation.

Mother's story
She had no problem being born. She was small and sleepy at first but she seemed fine and active. On her first day, she lost 200 grams (6 oz). I was concerned about getting enough food in her so I started breast-feeding her right away. She had such a small mouth that I also used a syringe to feed her. She was taking a good amount and everything was fine. On the third day, we started using a bottle with breast milk to get more nourishment to her. During the second feeding with a bottle her face went grey, she slumped over and became droopy. She was not breathing, so I patted her back and she came back to normal. After that she became lethargic and sleepy. That was the start of it all. The nurses took her back to the nursery and observed her. She had been lying there for 3 hours without any problem. We fed her again by having her father hold her upright while I held the bottle in her mouth. She took gulps and was sucking down strongly. Suddenly she stopped drinking and stopped breathing. That was the second episode. Something was wrong and we determined that she needed to go to the neonatal intensive care unit and put on a monitor.

After one of these episodes, she became even sleepier than usual. I was concerned if she was getting enough food because she was too sleepy to eat. After the first episode, she went 8 hours without a full meal. If I would try to feed her, she would have an episode and fall asleep. She will take milk from a bottle and be doing fine. Then at a certain point she stops sucking the bottle. She gets a look on her face like clamping down, wincing and pursing her lips and looses all energy. Where she had been active before, now she stays still. In just a few seconds, her oxygen goes down. Her face gets pale and then grey and purple especially at the eyes and lips and forehead and her chest stops moving. I know now that is from falling oxygen saturation in the blood. Once she has an episode she will often be too sleepy to eat. It is hard to arouse her from that sleep. That is the typical 'desaturation' episode. She has had two episodes outside of a feeding cycle. We now monitor her respiratory rate and that can tell us if an episode is coming.

The doctors have failed to identify any likely cause for the episodes. None of the tests showed anything definitive. They put a camera in her throat and there was no problem. An ultrasound of brain and heart was normal. An X-ray of the upper gastrointestinal area was fine and the reflux probe showed nothing. Even the bronchoscopy done when she was two weeks old was normal. She had a barium swallow, which showed she aspirated a bit of the liquid given to her. The test was tried again with thickened liquid and that did not happen. She did not go into an episode. Since then, we have been using thickened breast milk and she has had fewer episodes. The theory became that she was aspirating while eating and that caused the episodes but later the doctors doubted that is the issue.

The pregnancy was uneventful. There were no physical problems but I just felt a lot more tired. I had to take long naps because I did not have the energy. I got stressed and impatient more easily. Towards the end of the last half I had a lot of strong anger come up about my parents just as it used to. It came out of nowhere. It was more intense and continuous than any time in recent years. I felt helpless and victimised. There was nothing I could do to strike back. My regular remedy helped me when that happened.

Two dreams occurred near the end of my pregnancy. In each, I felt that I was having someone else's dream. There was a guy and I confronted him because he had lied to me. I couldn't trust him. In another dream I had gone back in time. In New York City's central park there was a famous baseball field. It was an historical site and I was connected to it somehow in a powerful way. I was feeling a lot of nostalgia. There was a group of people there like a reunion. It was as if years earlier we had been in war together or some other intense situation and it was great meeting up again. The feeling was like we had shared some intense experience or an intense difficult situation and we had to survive together. We had to flee the country because of the danger that we were in. Maybe we had been exiled together. There was a sense that we had been clinging together, sticking together and protecting each other. It was life and death and we were trying to survive.

A few days before I went in the hospital for the caesarean section I started to realise what was going to happen. I pictured myself lying on the operating table awake and someone cutting into my belly. For two days that kept running through my mind. I had read what the experience was like. You feel tugging, pulling and movement. That idea of lying there and knowing that someone was cutting into me freaked me out. When this happens I am likely to pass out. This was strange because I had already had a caesarean section for my first child and I had not had these kinds of thoughts or any worry. I kept having the image of lying there and feeling someone pulling at my insides, pulling me apart and tearing open my body while I knew what was going on. Talking about it now makes me feel woozy. In my imagination, I felt that scary sensation of pulling and tugging. I was being cut open and having someone doing that to me. It was happening but I was not feeling anything. I had all those sensations without the pain. My brain understood what was going on but I was disconnected from it. It made me feel nauseous and queasy and disconnected. My brain can't process that on a sensory level. I was repulsed and afraid. I wanted to run away but I was helpless. It was like watching a horror movie. I had no control and that is a disturbing feeling.

Even now, I feel the blood rush to my face and I am getting lightheaded. I am panicked right now like I am feeling that tugging. Someone is in there pulling and I don't know what that person is doing. Fear grips my stomach and my heart is racing. I wanted to sit down and take breaths because I am feeling weak right now. My body is in crisis mode and I will faint. Everything is rushing down from head and arms to my stomach. I am seeing the intestine pulled on. They are pulling me apart. Someone is pulling pieces of me off. I am getting disconnected. Pieces of me are ripped off from my insides and everything would fall apart. That is what is holding me together. Blood is gushing down and out. They are taking what is holding me together and yanking it out. A part of me is leaving my body that should be left in there. It is being ripped out. Someone rips it open and all the blood will go gushing out. I will be drained and die. They are pulling and pulling until finally something will rip. I tear and the blood is gushing out. Some of the organs will come out. I have the feeling of having myself pulled out of me. I am having a part of my body that I need pulled out. It is terrifying and I am helpless. There is nothing I can do.

Then there was pulling and tugging and right at my center. All my soft vulnerable stuff is there and they are yanking at me. It is not just a part of my body: it is me. They are pulling pieces out. There is something that they are pulling like an intestine but also something attached to my abdominal wall. I feel so out of control. I am disconnected. I am not me anymore. I felt as if I am half dead. I am still alive and feeling things but a part of me is not part of me anymore. It is like having my body cut in half. I have lost half of my body. When there is pulling and tugging I am not really feeling the pain of it. I am disconnected from it. I just have the sensation that they are doing it. I am not really there. It is as if I am watching someone else. I am not in my own body anymore. I have been disconnected from my body. It is as if I am floating in helplessness. My consciousness is floating there but I am not connected. There is a grey cloud right above my body and that is me. That is all I am. My brain is there and I am there watching but I am not able to do anything. I can't move my legs. I can't do anything.

Analysis
The problem with this newborn was her sudden ceasing to breath. No definitive aetiology or physiological reason was determined, although some aspiration was observed. In the absence of any other cause, this was thought to be the reason for her apnoea.

The most peculiar aspect to this case was the change in the mother's symptoms near the end of the pregnancy and most distinctively during the two days before the scheduled delivery. For many years, the mother responded extremely well to Androctonus. During the pregnancy, there were occasions during which her usual symptoms surfaced and a dose of Androctonus resolved the problems. Over the years the potencies used ranged from 200c-10M.

Under these circumstances, it might be supposed that the newborn would require the same remedy. Androctonus, as is true of the entire homeopathic group of spiders, can display symptoms of suffocation and dyspnoea. What is missing as support for that idea is any distinctive symptomatic connection from the child to the mother's state.

Near the end of the pregnancy, the mother had two dreams, which were distinctive in that she felt as if she were having someone else's dream. They felt unfamiliar to her, thereby presenting the first clue that she was experiencing some other state than her familiar one. Two days before the delivery, she begins to have frightening thoughts and imaginations, very different than she had ever had before. Despite having had a successful caesarean section several years earlier, her behaviour is as if she has never had that experience before. This is another clue supporting the idea that she is not in her usual state, but is acting as if she is someone else – someone who has never experienced the operation before; someone who has dreams of having been in a frightening and dangerous situation like a war. What is apparent is a change in the mother's symptoms away from her usual symptom pattern and the presentation of a different picture.

Where is this other set of symptoms coming from? Rather than the mother's state influencing the child's, it is most likely that the child's state must be influencing her. The change from one state, as evidenced by one symptom pattern to another distinct pattern, indicates that a new and different remedy is needed. This can happen to any patient at any time. During pregnancy, this change in the mother is typically from the influence of the child *in utero* and her state.

Having seen that the mother is exhibiting new symptoms in the last days of pregnancy, what remedy do they indicate for the newborn with episodic apnoea? The most common remedy for neonatal asphyxia is Opium, especially in light of anaesthesia during delivery or the shock of the birth process. Two relevant rubrics are:

- Respiration, Asphyxia or suffocation in the newborn infant.
- Mind, Ailments from shock.

Choice of remedy

Looking at the mother's dreams, there is a fear of having been in a dangerous, life-threatening situation, such as war. The rubrics that come to mind are:

- Mind, Ailments from fright.
- Mind, Fear of impending death.
- Mind, Dreams of war.

Furthermore, her imaginations are fearful and of being cut open but not feeling the pain. These symptoms are indicated by:

- Generalities, Painlessness of complaints usually painful.
- Generalities, Anaesthesia and insensibility.

She has fearful thoughts and describes the cutting and trauma that she imagines as her body being in crisis and she will faint as shown with:

- Generalities, Fainting from fright.
- Generalities, Unconsciousness from the shock in injury.

She experiences a sensation of dissociation to what is happening to her, that she is not in her body anymore. She feels as if she is hovering over her own body watching it, described as:

- Mind, Delusions, is floating in air.

All of these sensations, feelings and thoughts combined with the neonatal asphyxia episodes point to Opium as a remedy for the infant. She was given Opium 200c on day 14 of her young life.

Follow up
The child had minimal response to the remedy. She continued to have desaturation episodes but with a slight decrease in frequency and intensity the first few days after the remedy. The episodes were still followed by sleepiness. She was gaining weight and within three days after the remedy, she had almost returned to her birth weight. Another dose of Opium 200 was given on day 21. Again there was a small response, which only lasted a few days.

Review
Despite the indications, the response to the two doses of Opium was not enough to warrant continuation of that remedy. A reassessment of the case was needed. The most intense aspect was not the dreams, which occurred several months prior to the end of the pregnancy. They served to indicate that another state was developing. However, the most peculiar aspect of the case was the mother's fear during the two days prior to the caesarean section. Despite having had the same operation quite successfully previously, her experience now was as if it was unknown and terrifying. Her fears and imaginations were so real to her that she became dizzy and upset merely talking about them during the interview, several weeks after they occurred. Highest consideration was now given to the most outstanding feature of these fears and sensations. Granted, she still had the lack of pain for painful events and the sensation of flying. They were not, however, the key and most peculiar aspect.

The key sensation the mother experienced during her imagination about the upcoming caesarean section is the feeling of being cut open, pulled apart and something important being pulled out. It is not just a part of her that is being pulled and ripped out. A part of her body that should remain there is being ripped out and there is blood all around. She feels that she is being pulled; she feels as if she is half, because she has been cut into two. She is not herself anymore because part has been cut out, being disconnected from herself. She has lost half of herself. The most prevalent sensation throughout her fears is that of being cut, cut in two, being disconnected and ripped apart.

From her visual imagery, it is not difficult to perceive the connection to a real caesarean section. That is exactly what happens – the body is cut open and the child is removed. There are two where before there was one. This vivid account of her fears and their relation to the birthing process she was about to undergo, lead me to consider the 2nd row of the periodic table.

Whether the child is born this way or in the normal process, there comes a moment when the child becomes completely and totally disconnected from the mother. The cutting of the umbilical cord makes the final disconnection. The theme of cutting, separating into two and removing part of her to make her half clearly indicates the remedy. Fluoric acid has to do with the cutting to separate completely. Though there are not many rubrics that specifically represent this, there are some which indicate the theme of separation between family members, such as:

- Mind, Delusions, she must drive children out of the house.
- Mind, Aversion to family members.

The child was given Fluoric acid 200c on day 25 of her life.

Follow up
Within 36 hours of the remedy, she was having significantly fewer de-saturation episodes and they were of much less intensity than before. She was more alert, focused and engaged with the surroundings. Within a week after the remedy, she would go whole days without episodes. She had improved enough to allow her to be discharged from the hospital. After over a month in the hospital, at age 34 days, her mother and father took their child home. After returning home, she had a few mild episodes and one larger one but the parents were able to get her out of them easily.

She continued to be more active with kicking and moving. Sometimes she would be wide awake and looking all around her. She slept a lot and woke to eat. After coming home, she had a great increase in volume of milk, almost doubling her intake, indicating a growth spurt. She was even able to nurse for a while. She very aggressively wanted to eat. She took milk seven times a day.

The mother reports, 'I am connected to her but something is missing. I am not as connected as I was the other child. With him immediately I was holding him all the time and nursing him directly. As soon as he was born he was a part of me very quickly. That has happened with her but not as complete. I would go away when she was in the hospital and there was that physical distance from her. It interfered with the total bonding. I am bonded but not as completely. She is not as completely inside me every moment. I don't always feel her there. She is bonded with me. She knows me and she knows and recognises me. She looks at me and into my eyes.

I felt that she is comfortable with me. When she would look I didn't feel like she was really seeing me as much. She was not focusing on anything as much.'

With her increase in growth, another dose of Fluoric acid 200c was given. Over the ensuing weeks, she would have many days in a row without episodes. Occasionally, she would look like she would start to have one but would not go into it. At about two months of age, she had a cold for several days with snuffles and sniffles. Her mother reported that the child had been more tired. A few days prior, her milk intake increased 50% and she was eating every two hours. The Fluoric acid 200c was repeated. She responded with several episodes in the following 24 hours and then no more after that. The congestion resolved. Within a week she weighed 3.7 kg (8 lbs 5 oz) and measured 53 cm (21 in).

At three months of age, the desaturation episodes occurred only rarely and were very mild. The mother reports that the child responds and interacts and is interested in the surroundings. She is very alert and engaged. The mother's connection to the child is much better. She is beginning to 'perceive her presence even when I am not with her. That is happening more and more.'

Further comments

This case is instructive for several reasons. Firstly, it is a good example of the child's state exerting influence on the mother. It could also be said that the mother and child, together went to the Fluoric acid state. However, after delivery, the mother never needed Fluoric acid and has returned to her usual remedy.

The other important point of this case is the difference between prescribing on usual symptoms and going deeply into the vital sensation. Assessing the case initially, Opium seemed like a good choice, supported as it was with symptoms, rubrics, keynotes and experience with the remedy. That choice, however, overlooked the theme and most important peculiar of the case – the ideas of separation and cutting. This experience highlights that keynotes and rubrics, no matter how accurate, cannot make up for excluding the most peculiar aspect of a case.

8

THE CHILD'S ENVIRONMENT

The child lives in a world made up of other people, events and changes; all of which reflect and affect the child. As mentioned in previous chapters, stressful events in a child's life can exacerbate symptoms, use up the energy of the remedy dose or even imprint a new state on the child, necessitating a different remedy. Whereas many usual childhood events such as teething, starting school or having a new sibling born into the family, are well known to have an impact on children, there are other less well-known events that also have an influence. Investigation into all of these areas provides information useful to understanding his world.

Nature versus nurture

Long and heated has been the debate on whether a person's character and life is more under the influence of his inherent nature or of the environment he finds himself in. Is it nature or nurture that is of most importance to development? As discussed in chapter four, most now agree that the two are intertwined and interrelated, each playing a part in harmonious interaction. Homeopaths view this matter in a slightly different way. Another player in the equation determines both the nature and nurture – the energy state.

A basic tenet of homeopathic philosophy is that the inner dynamic state, what here is called the energy field or energy state, determines everything about the person. His physical body, emotions, character, mental faculties, interests, desires and aversions are all related to his inner state. Consequently, all aspects of a person's life resulting from these qualities are indirectly determined by the inner state. This includes the relationships a person forms, the profession pursued, the choices about his direction in life and the things that happen to him. Even accidents or events seemingly well outside a person's jurisdiction are influenced by his inner state. We know that 'the brick always falls on the head of the Arnica patient.' Whatever event occurs, the person's reaction to it and what it means to him will likewise be determined by his state of being. Suffice it to say, the state inside dictates what goes on in the outside environment.

Homeopaths frequently witness the changes, often very dramatic ones, which a patient makes in his life as he becomes healthier under the remedies' influence. Jobs are changed, goals are realised, new friendships are formed and destructive influences are abandoned. Good health does not stop at the skin; it radiates to encompass everything about the person's life and environment.

Causa occasionalis

Having said that, things are a bit different with children. The principle is the same; the reality is different. As adults get better, they can change their environment. They can get a better job, leave a bad relationship, improve their eating habits or make any other change. In other words, as they get healthier, they have the mental and emotional strength to remove what Hahnemann refers to as sustaining causes or 'causa occasionalis' – those aspects of their life and environment that reflected and sustained their ill health.

No matter how healthy they get, children do not have that possibility. They are dependent on the existing environment and consequently have far less volitional control over it. A child's sickness can be the repository and effect of the problems in the household, the parent's relationship or the lifestyle of the family. Until or unless those adverse and unhealthy situations resolve, the child will be constantly affected by their influence. These sustaining causes are a constant stress, which the child must perpetually use his energy to cope with.

Certainly an unhealthy child has an impact on the family, his schoolmates and friends, often causing stress or disturbance. When his health improves, the whole dynamic of the family or classroom can change for the better. What a child cannot do in the same way as an adult, is to leave a situation or remove himself from adverse or unhealthy environmental influences that he cannot change. This is an important difference to consider when treating children. As healthy as the child can get under the homeopathic treatment, he can never completely rise above the health of the family of which he is part.

What does that mean to the homeopath? It could mean that the correct remedy does not seem to act as thoroughly or the dose does not last as long as expected. It could also mean that the homeopath doubts his remedy selection and is tempted to switch to another in the hopes of finding one that will work more dramatically. It is important to remember that the remedy is simply energy. When that energy is occupied doing one task, it is not available for another. In practice that means that the energy of the remedy being used to assist the child to cope with daily stressful influences will not be available to support as much progress in healing. Consequently, relapses are more frequent, requiring that doses are repeated more often than customary.

Aetiology and vulnerability

Not only do children lack the prospect of leaving stressful environments, they are also more malleable, more susceptible to influences. This is another difference between adults and children. In general, they have not developed the resilience, stability, strength or coping mechanisms to withstand influences or compensate for them.

The child psychologist and psychotherapist Dr. Haim Ginott (1922–1973) is reputed to have said:

'Children are like wet cement. Whatever falls on them makes an impression.'

This is not a flaw in children. As we will discuss in the next chapter, there are very important developmental reasons for this receptivity to sensory and external influences without which normal neural maturation would not be possible. Nonetheless, being aware of their susceptibility and the influences they are exposed to gives the homeopath a great deal of useful information about the child and what may be contributing to his ailments.

For example, even full-term and healthy newborns do not have the ability to regulate their temperature and consequently are completely dependent on their environment for maintenance of a constant body temperature. This compounded the problem for the child suffering from coeliac disease in chapter seven. Newborns may not be able to maintain their body temperature if the environment is too cold. Being unable to maintain the critical balance between internal heat production and heat loss, they have a far narrower range of environmental temperatures and can overheat or suffer critical heat loss very easily. Whereas an adult can comfortably accommodate a slightly cool room, the newborn might sustain significant heat loss.

It is not merely physical and physiological functions that are less resilient in the young than in adults. The child's emotional and mental functions also demonstrate the vulnerability and susceptibility to outside influences. From the classic scenario of a young child being afraid of the dark to the fright from witnessing his mother disappear behind a door; a child's reactions clearly reveal his sensitivity. The functional development of his brain (as described in chapter four) plays a primary role in how the child experiences these events and what they mean to him.

For this reason aetiologies, or as homeopaths refer to them, 'never well since' events are more important to consider than in adults. For children, influences are more often true aetiologies whereas in adults a stress or influence more typically activates pre-existing weaknesses from their constitutional state.

Most diseases in children have an emotional component or aetiology. The younger the child, the more true this is. However, the younger the child, the more difficult it is to perceive what that emotional aspect is. Consider the pre-verbal child. They have no words to express their emotions. The various modulations of their cries are all that is available for their verbal communication. Notably distinguishable by their mother into an array of different needs and messages, a child's cry is still a very limited means of communication, especially of the nuances of emotional distress. What they cannot express in words, they express through their body as symptoms. This is not to say that a child's symptoms are psychosomatic. Those fevers are real; that ear infection is real; the colic, rash, asthma and vomiting are all very real. Without emotional perception or vocabulary at their disposal, this is a way of communicating their inner state.

For a similar reason, a category called 'childhood illness' which a child can 'out grow' has been designated. As the child grows, the abilities resulting from emotional and mental maturation take over what the body used to have to do. The older child has the verbally capability to express distress, emotional pain or unhappiness. From a larger perspective, the child is learning and developing mechanisms of inner protection and coping to help maintain his healthy state in the face of various emotional and physical stresses in a way similar to the way a newborn develops thermoregulation to be able to cope with a large world of widely fluctuating temperatures.

When regarding any symptom, we should always be asking ourselves, 'What is the child's body communicating about his inner state?' Putting together the pieces of external influences and events, specific physical symptoms, age of the child's development and parental influence are necessary to decipher what is being expressed.

Adoption

The state of the mother during pregnancy plays a central role in determining a child's health and allowing us to discover his inner state. How should the homeopath approach the situation where that information is not available, such as with the adopted child? Occasionally access to the prenatal and birth records and even the birth mother is available. Most often, however, this information about the adopted child is not known. Sometimes information about the pre-adoption circumstances is unknown. I treat several young girls adopted from China in addition to several children from Russia and other eastern European countries. Details of their life in the orphanage remain unspecified.

Suffice it to say, many orphanages in China, Asia, Central Europe, Russia and other countries are not affluent enough to be as supportive of their children as one would hope. Often overcrowding, an impoverished environment, lack of emotional care and support, inadequate educational or medical facilities can contribute to a difficult pre-adoption life. Though the specifics are not known, these early experiences have a tremendous impact on the child. For these girls and many other adopted children, all we can know with certainty are the symptoms the child displays. Careful homeopathic prescribing has a powerful effect on helping the child recover from these early stressful influences.

Family dynamics: parents, siblings, extended family members

The child is in an environment populated by other family members and care-takers each of which forms a relationship to him, thereby creating an impact on each other. Influences do not stop there. The family, as an entity in itself, is composed of a web of interactions and influences between all family members, all of which play their part in forming the environment the child experiences. In that mix, one sick child will send a ripple of disturbing influences throughout the entire family. It is not just that illness in the family affects all members. When ill, a child's state of being is intensified, thereby intensifying the inner states of all other people in the family, which then affect each other more intensely.

For example, in a family of five, the youngest child, age four, develops a cough and fever in the late afternoon. By bedtime, the child is cranky, restless and coughing. He wants to be held and rocked. The cough persists throughout the night, keeping the mother awake, while she holds him upright pacing the floor. Many parents will recognise this scenario. Even if the child recovers the next day, now the mother is stressed from being worried and sleep deprived. Her temper is shorter the next day. Try as she might to function normally, she exhibits less patience with the other children and her husband. The stability, safety and predict-ability of the household have been disturbed. The other two children will react to this situation in different ways depending on their inner state, but react they will.

The children sense that their mother is irritable and their younger sibling is acting differently too. What is going on? When will everything be restored to normal? What has gone wrong? Did they do anything wrong? These and many other conscious and unconscious thoughts pass through their minds. Funda-mentally, their stress is the disturbance to the stability of the household. Their stress may manifest as the development of symptoms. The father comes home to an exhausted wife, one cranky feverish coughing child and two others feeling uneasy, out of sorts and on their way to manifesting their particular array of symptoms and behaviours. Is it any wonder that as the days pass he, too, may soon show signs of illness? With three sick children and a husband who is begin-ning to feel the effects of this stress, mother now succumbs to the effects of her caring for the other family members. With so much resting on her shoulders, she cannot afford to be ill so she forces herself to carry on her duties despite feeling so poorly. No wonder her illness lasts much longer than anyone else's. I call this the 'family meltdown'.

After a few days, the originally ill child will be feeling better, but in his wake are the ravages of a stressed household. With everyone around him in some stage of illness, it is likely that he will relapse within weeks. How many times do we hear of a cold or flu passing from one family member to another in sequence, commonly attributed to the passing of germs? It is not necessarily the germs. More likely any illness is due to the stress that gets passed around resulting in increased susceptibility to the existing germs in the environment.

When one member of the family is treated homeopathically, the entire family benefits. Even one in the group being better able to get well and stay well assists to break the family meltdown cycle described above. When additional family members are also treated, even more benefit is derived as each member has a healthier relationship with the others. A tendency to family meltdown turns into a tendency to family unity, enjoyment and happiness.

Naturally there will always be the normal stage of growth and development which can result in age-appropriate tensions or challenges within the family. However when treated with homeopathy, those stages are met with greater strength and resilience.

What can we as homeopaths do to assist our child patient? I encourage parents to consider having as many of the family members treated as possible by explaining just what I have written above to the parents. Once aware of these dynamics, most parents see them for themselves. When treating only one child in the family, I still enquire into the other family members and family dynamics, stresses and events that have occurred.

School, friends and social development

For the first years of a child's life, his world is centred in the home with his parents and family. As he grows, his world enlarges to include other people and places. This socialisation usually occurs at about four to five years old, after the child has established his sense of safety, security and identity within the home and family. Too early introduction into the wider world before the home is a stable and safe place can be very frightening to the child. Too late an entrance into the social world can delay the child's social maturation.

Talking to school aged children will centre on what is important to them; usually their friends, school, siblings, parents and after school activities. On the canvas of those topics a child's inner state paints itself. To understand their state, search beneath the specific topics and look for their feelings, experience, reactions and thoughts.

Orthodontic braces

Many children have orthodontic braces put on their teeth for anywhere from one to three years, to correct malocclusions or other structural dental problems (see figure 8.1). Braces move each tooth in a particular direction through the use of force created by the metal bands and wires on the teeth acting on the periodontal ligament. Additionally the bone in which the teeth are rooted undergoes structural changes and remodelling as a result of effects on the periodontal blood supply. As the teeth move, frequent readjustments to the orthodontic apparatus are required, usually every six to eight weeks. Bone is absorbed, and reformed, blood supply is altered and there is strain on the sensitive tooth ligaments. Suffice it to say, this is not a painless ordeal. Significant discomfort or even frank pain often occurs for the first several months and then for the several days after each readjustment during the first year. This chronic level of dental pain may have an impact on the action of the remedy. Typically, additional doses are required during the first year of orthodontic treatment.

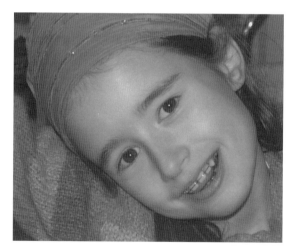

Figure 8.1 Child wearing orthodontic brace.

Accidents

Accidents are a frequent part of life. I recall an incident years ago involving a mother who brought her young son to me for his annual back-to-school physical examination. She provided me with the usual form to fill in about the child's medical history and the examination. She had already filled in her section about the child, including the questions , 'Accidents?' and 'Please explain'. To the first, she answered 'No.' and to the second she replied 'Sheer luck!'

How should a homeopath handle accidents during a child's constitutional treatment? We should do what we always do: take the case and find the correct remedy. Not everyone who bruises themselves needs Arnica montana. Many situations involving accidents are better treated with the person's constitutional remedy. Only a full survey of the patient and the situation will reveal what remedy is needed.

Immunisations

Most parents have questions about immunisations. It is incumbent on the homeopath to answer their questions and address their fears, helping the parents understand many of the fallacies, incorrect assumptions and mis-information about immunisations, enabling them to make a more informed choice. Though most of the information in this section is known to homeopaths, it may serve to help explain the topic to parents.

It is common for parents to regard immunisations as the only way to protect their child. They need to understand that not giving immunisations does not mean the child is without protection. Treating with homeopathy gives better protection and this section outlines ways of explaining these concepts to the parents.

Immunisations use a small amount of a disease toxin or the protein segment or the entire body of a disease-causing micro-organism, sometimes as a live virus. This foreign substance is introduced into the body of the child. In the past polio was administered orally. Today, all immunisations are injected, bypassing many of the body's natural defences, such as skin, nasal and throat mucus. The benefits of this procedure are thought to come from the response the body makes to these injected foreign substances. As a reaction to most foreign proteins and many toxins, the body's immune system mounts an immunological response.

The immune system and its functions are extremely intricate and complex. It is composed of a wide range of organs including spleen, bone marrow, thymus, hundreds of lymph nodes, miles of lymph channels, a variety of cells such as macrophages, neutrophils, eosinophils, lymphocytes and others, antibodies of an almost infinite variety, a cascade of dozens of chemicals such as histamine, bradykinin, specific proteins called complements and others, all acting in concert with each other. There are two main branches of the immune system; one is for fighting acute infections and produces antibodies, and the other protects against long-term viruses and aberrant cells like cancer. The function of the immune system is of such complexity that much of it is still not understood, despite decades of intensive research.

From the first mention of immunity by Thucydides during a plague in Athens in 430 BC, who observed resistance to a second infection of the same disease, until today, there has been much effort to learn about these physical phenomena. Edward Jenner (1749-1823) made the first immunisation for smallpox, then called vaccination because of his use of cows in the making of the treatment (the Latin for cow being *vaccus*). Now there are vaccines for tetanus, diphtheria, whooping cough (pertussis), hepatitis A, hepatitis B, pneumococcus, hemophilus influenzae, measles, mumps, polio, rubella, varicella, herpes zoster, human papillomavirus, meningococcus and retrovirus. Following the full schedule of vaccines recommended by the USA's Centers for Disease Control[1] the programme starts with a hepatitis B vaccine at birth, followed by upwards of 48 additional vaccines by the time the child is six years old!

The premise on which immunisations are founded is that they will stimulate the person's own immune system to develop antibodies and other factors to confer permanent immunity against the selected disease. By exposing the person to a very small amount of the protein or actual infecting organism, his immune system function is inaugurated to develop life-long protection without making the person suffer the entire disease.

One very common misunderstanding about immunisations and 'allergy shots', a series of injections given over months, with the purpose of desensitizing a person to things they are allergic to such as dust, pollens and grasses, is that they are based on the same principles as homeopathy: that a small dose of the disease confers protection. Though on the surface there appears to be a similarity, nothing could be further from the truth. Homeopathy and immunisations do not work in the same way, nor do they have anything in common.

Immunisations are an artificial stimulation of the body's immune system through the introduction into the body of a foreign protein, micro-organisms or toxins. Though the amount of the substance is small, it is still present and measurable. Homeopathic remedies, however, are non-material, formed of and working on the energy level of a person. The use of immunisations does not match the symptoms of the disease to the symptoms of the treatment. The measles vaccine is given to prevent measles, despite no symptoms being present. Again, this is completely different than the fundamental premise of homeopathy, which is based on prescribing the simillimum based on the totality of symptoms. The homeopathic nosode Variolinum, made from smallpox, is a case in point. The homeopathic indications are the symptoms from cured cases which did not necessarily have smallpox, not the description or diagnosis of smallpox. The same is true of Tuberculinum, Diphtherinum, Pertussinum and others. Allergy shots are made up of a variety of particular substances that a person has shown immunological reaction to. There is no relationship between the nature of those reactions, the person's individualised symptoms and the substance diluted in the injections.

After being immunised, the body is forced to do something it would not be inclined to do if left on its own. If treatment were needed, the person would exhibit individualising symptoms to guide the doctor as to what treatment is needed. Furthermore, there is no individualisation; all children get the same immunisations. The essence of homeopathy is the acknowledgment of the individual expression each person has through the individualisation of treatment. Immunisations are the universal treatment of asymptomatic children by injecting them with a foreign substance to artificially force their bodies to function in an abnormal way.

The timing of immunisations is perplexing. Immunisations are supposed to work by activating the person's immune system through controlled exposure to a substance. Approximately 23 of the recommended childhood immunisations are given to the infant on or before he is six months old. At two months old seven are given all at once, two months later another six are given, and two months after that, six more are given at one time! This has always been an enigma to me. The infant's immune system is not active at birth; it is still in its nascent state just as are his heart, nervous system, eyes, teeth and bones and liver. The growing foetus does not have the need of its own functioning immune system in utero. It receives immunity from the mother through the placenta.

Once born, however, the situation changes and the infant is definitely going to need a fully functioning immune system. During the first six months of life, the immune system begins the long, complex process of maturation. While this is happening, immunity still comes from the mother through the breast milk. At the end of six months, the immune system is still far from completely matured; that will take several more years. It can, however, begin protecting the child. Concomitant with the child's immune system becoming increasingly functional, the maternally conferred immunity in the breast milk declines. Starting at birth, the infant's immune system increases strength while the maternal contribution to his immunity declines. The six-month mark is significant because that is the cross-over point. Up to that time, the mother's immunity gives the majority of the protection. After that, more immune protection is provided by the child's own immune system.

This being the case, what are the 23 immunisations given to children under the age of six months activating? There is no functional immune system to prompt into immune action. The immature, barely functional immune system can hardly be expected to respond appropriately, or even adequately to being bombarded by foreign substances that have bypassed the defence barriers by inoculation. We do not expect the infant to chew steak at two months, or run a race, recite a speech, operate a computer, calculate math problems or even tie his shoes. Yet, through immunisations, doctors expect his immune system to perform functions that it will not be capable of for many years. In fact, the very act of introducing such a demand on the immune system's carefully constructed complex cascade of developmental stages disrupts this process, sometimes irreparably and not infrequently wrecking havoc to the entire child.

Why do immunisations cause such a problem? Chapter four discussed the topic of developmental stages and the precision with which sequences of events unfold at just the right time and in just the right order. This applies to all aspects of the child, including the immune system. All immune organs and functions must blossom in a coordinated way, at just the right time, as the child matures. During the first five to six years of the child's life, his immune system undergoes the majority of this development. It will not be until after puberty that he will have a fully functional immune system that will offer protection for the rest of his life. This process works extremely well on its own to do what it is designed to do.

Immunisations try to improve on this natural development by shortening the process. Instead of the immune system developing in a coordinated way along a precise time line, the unnatural introduction of foreign protein and toxins by injection confronts the immature immune system with a challenge it is not ready for. Not only does the immune system respond in an inadequate way, there is confusion and disturbance in the entire maturation process. The same thing would happen if a two-year-old tried to lift 25 kg (55 lb), or was put into a high school class. It reminds me of the 'hurry up and learn' approach of children being put into schools at an earlier and earlier age. Right event; wrong time of life. When it comes to the attitude to children, our fast-paced, impatient culture has influenced people to such a degree that they cannot seem to wait for the normal processes of development; socially, mentally or immunologically. Confusion results.

Parents will ask how that can be so, since immunisations work to confer immunity against the diseases intended. A child immunised against measles will usually not contract it. Yes, the immune system, immature and partially functional as it is, will often, but not always, produce the desired antibodies. The unseen problem, the price, for forcing that function out of schedule is that the immune system becomes disordered; the normal development is disrupted. The incidence of childhood immune-related and other diseases such as asthma and arthritis has skyrocketed. For example, there is a 17-fold increase in childhood diabetes, from 1 in 7,100 children in 1950 to 1 in 400 today.[2]

Most susceptible to this immune disordering is the brain. Improper immune stimulation alters the brain's supportive glial cells function. Instead of assisting brain development, they release many toxic substances that damage brain cells and their interconnections, resulting in autism and other developmental problems. Prior to immunisations, autism was an extremely rare disorder. Today, one in 68 families has an autistic child and one out of every six children is classified as learning disabled.[2] Nothing can even begin to compensate for a normal child being damaged by immunisations. Yet the $1.5 billion (£972k, €1.1bn) paid out over the years by the US government through its Vaccine Injury Compensation Program[3] attests to the harm that vaccines can cause.[4] These are stunning statistics with devastating consequences.

In addition to forcing the immune system to function out of its desired schedule, there is a problem with bypassing the experience of childhood diseases in the first place. As mentioned, the immune system maturation is a well-orchestrated, complex process occurring over many years. In the same way, education of a child requires many years of schooling, each year systematically and progressively building on what was learned in previous years. Periodic testing is used not only to assess what a child has learned, but also to challenge, stimulate and motivate the child to develop. Such is it with immune development. Challenges are needed to activate the immune system, building its inner mechanisms of protection and function. In fact, without such challenges at just the right time in the early stages of development, the immune system will be deficient for the rest of the child's life, in similar fashion to a child that does not learn to read by age six to ten years, will usually be illiterate to some degree for the rest of his life. The exposure to any of the group of childhood infectious illness at just the right time in childhood provides exactly the stimulating challenge the child's immune system needs to mature in a fully functional and efficient way. Stimulation to the immune system with immunisations does not provide the same positive effect for all the reasons described above; it bypasses normal defence barriers; it is given at the wrong time; forces the immune system to act in a way it is not developed enough to do; disorders the normal maturation process.

The consequences of these disruptions and improper maturation may not show up for years. It is this delay in the manifestation of immune system development disruption and damage that makes it hard for the conventional medical world to see a connection between a childhood immunisation and an immune malfunction in middle age. What are the long-term consequences of tampering with a developing immune system? Any immune malfunction at any time in life can occur. This is a very serious situation. The immune system is not just for fighting infections; it has been implicated in a variety of chronic diseases such as arteriosclerosis, thyroiditis, arthritis, cancer, a whole variety of auto-immune diseases and many other chronic afflictions. Having mumps as a four-year-old trains the immune system, laying the foundation for proper working that will later protect against these kinds of chronic illnesses that are the consequence of immune malfunction.

Many parents ask, 'If not immunisations, then what?' Though we are many decades from a life in which children were crippled from polio, died from pertussis or diphtheria or became blind after measles, the memory and fear are still alive. Yes, certainly it is easy to understand why there has been the drive for finding a way to avoid having children exposed to these dangers.

Before addressing this question, a little historical information will help put these fears in perspective, and understand what the dangers really are. The dramatic decline or elimination of infectious childhood diseases is universally credited to the widespread use of immunisation. So strongly has this idea been put across that parents accept it without question and it becomes an almost impenetrable barrier beyond which it is fearful to venture. For many of the most frightening diseases such as measles, polio, diphtheria and pertussis, this is not what actually happened. In each case, the incidence and mortality of the disease had declined sharply *before* immunisations were used. Increased nutrition, a better standard of living, cleaner water, better sewage removal and dramatic improvements in sanitation and hygiene were solely responsible for the great reductions in these diseases. For example, in 1920, there were 7575 deaths from measles in USA.[5] By 1963, the year before measles vaccine was used, that number was already reduced to 100. Still the conventional medical world, many government agencies and immunisation manufacturers insist that the decline in incidence and death from measles began only after immunisation. To prevent these remaining incidences, now millions of children are vaccinated, many thousands of whom will become brain damaged, learning disabled or autistic. It is not even possible to determine what health problems the rest will suffer later in life.

In addition to claiming full credit for saving children from the ravages of childhood illness, immunisation proponents attest to their complete safety citing medical research studies as firm evidence. Doctors make decisions about treatment, disease progress, and likely outcomes based on published medical research, the bedrock on which medical science is based. Medical research is assumed to be a completely independent, purely science inquiry to objectively evaluate various treatments, drugs and procedures.

At least in the field of immunisations, that is very far from the truth. A great majority of studies that conclusively promote immunisations are funded by the companies who make the vaccines or by doctors who receive a salary from those companies. These conflicts of interests are rarely disclosed. With vaccinations being a multi-billion dollar industry, these studies can hardly be considered objective scientific work. All of them come to the conclusion that immunisations are not only safe and effective but essential for a child's welfare. Furthermore, long-term safety of immunisations is assured but there is barely any medical research into the long-term effects of vaccines or their link to chronic immune related disorders. For example, the initial studies investigating the hepatitis vaccine for newborns claimed there are no adverse effects. However, they only evaluated infants for the first three months after inoculation. Any neurological or developmental problems occurring in a child on the fourth month would not be counted as an immunisation related problem. Comparing the incidence of chronic diseases between groups of children or adults who have been immunised and those who were not has also not been done.

Being aware of the spurious nature of some of the most unquestioned tenets of immunisation, helps put the issue of immunisations on a more realistic perspective. There is still the question of 'If not immunisations, then what?' The question of using immunisations is not one of protecting the child or not. Naturally, it is assumed that everyone wants his or her child protected. The real question is what is the best way to give the child the optimum protection. This is more than a rephrasing of the same issue: it is a different question altogether. The first presupposes that immunisations are the only way to protect a child from risk of communicable diseases, without which the child is in constant risk. The second asks which of several ways available will do the best job, giving the best results.

Homeopathy can provide that protection. The parents should know that it is not precisely accurate to think that it is the homeopathic remedy that gives the protection. What homeopathy does is to clear the way for the child to be so healthy that he is not susceptible to infections, whether colds, polio, tuberculosis, whooping cough, diphtheria, hepatitis or any other. It is the child's own natural and proper immune function, working the way it was designed to work that gives the maximum protection. It is only a sick child that is susceptible to these contagious diseases. It is most helpful if you can get the parents to understand one basic tenet of homeopathy – a child is not sick because he has an infectious ailment; he gets an infectious ailment because he is sick. Homeopathy makes sure he is not sick.

Immunising one's child has been such an integral, unquestioned precept of modern medicine that it is sometimes very frightening for parents to refrain from immunising their child. Naturally, the parents want to do what is best for their child. Even after having studied the issue from the increasing volume of articles, books and reports about the dangers, it remains a tremendously difficult decision for many parents, fraught with anxiety. No one can make that decision for them. You can provide information, encourage the parents to investigate for themselves and answer questions but ultimately, the parents must decide.

Final comments

All patients are influenced by and also influence their environment of people, events and situations. Investigating these areas is fruitful for any patient. In children's cases, however, they can play an even more important role in understanding the child. Being aware of ongoing stressful situations or family dynamics that the child cannot change will help to understand the child and give special insight in how to manage the case after the first prescription.

References

1   Centers for Disease Control and Prevention (Accessed December 16th 2009)
2   Miller D (Jr). A User Friendly Vaccination Schedule. 2004 Available online at LewRockwell.com Website http://tinyurl.com/63l3d (Accessed 16th December 2009)
3   National Vaccine Injury Compensation Program (VICP) Information available at HRSA.gov/vaccinecompensation (Accessed 16th December 2009)
4   Levin M. Vaccine Injury Claims face grueling fight, Los Angeles Times November 29th 2004. Available online at http://tinyurl.com/yezutr3 (Accessed 16th December 2009)
5   NIH/NIAD Emerging and Re-emerging Infectious Diseases Website. Available online at http://tinyurl.com/54mn2. Also see: United States Centers for Disease Control Morbidity and Mortality Weekly Reports Web site http://www.cdc.gov/mmwr (Accessed 16th December 2009)

9

PARENTS

The deputised parent

One of the most pleasant and rewarding aspects of treating children is working together with their parents for the benefit of the child. Homeopathy is not simply a treatment or medical system in which patients present themselves to the doctor who then fixes their problem, after which they go home again. Homeopathy is a cooperative effort using techniques and medicinal substances based on a philosophical perspective of life and healing.

From that perspective, it is essential to involve the parents in the treatment of their child. Making allies of the parents is extremely helpful, and in some cases indispensable, to do a good job for the child. Most parents, even the most knowledgeable, benefit from further education from the homeopath. I make it a point to spend quite a bit of time explaining to parents the basic viewpoints of homeopathy; how we look at health and disease, how we take into consideration the whole child not just isolated symptoms, what to expect from treatment, about return of old symptoms and how the remedy will act. Most importantly, I help the parent understand their child better and develop the skills to observe their child from the viewpoint of homeopathy. I call this process 'deputising the parent', further emphasising the team effort involved when treating children.

The education of parents is an ongoing process, each visit proving an opportunity to add a little more information, answer the questions at hand and continue to highlight details about the child and his development. I also inform parents what characteristics, developmental milestones or symptoms to watch for and what situations may be especially stressful on the child, given the remedy that he takes.

Guiding the parent this way by broadening their perspective on life through the basic ideas of homeopathy yields tremendous advantages. Firstly, a knowledgeable parent is better able to observe and report useful symptoms and characteristics to the homeopath, which in turn greatly helps the child. Secondly, parents have a more thorough understanding of their child, being better able to comprehend what the child's behaviour, physical symptoms and actions are communicating about his inner world. This opens a whole new level of understanding and empathetic connection, allowing a closer and more intimate bond to grow between parent and child. It is thrilling to witness that happen and be a part of it.

The value of educating and deputising parents becomes evident by reading the personal experience of one of my patients, Rachel Lipman Mostow. As a patient herself and the mother of four children treated with homeopathy, she is in a good position to describe what it is like for her to have the team approach in homeopathy.

Case 9.1   A parent's perspective

'Before I discovered homeopathic medicine for my children, I thought I knew how to take care of their health: I waited for them to become sick, then took them to the doctor to get medicine to cure the symptoms. Coughing, sneezing and fever were the enemy, and the doctor had a medicine for each one. Becoming a 'homeopathic parent' taught me how to stop looking at individual symptoms and start observing my whole child.

My road to homeopathy came from what I considered a life or death situation: my son's asthma had reached a crisis state. When my son, Ari, developed asthma as a baby, I took him to the top paediatric asthma specialist in the city. Although Ari wasn't allergic to anything and we couldn't find an underlying cause for his asthma, his attacks became more frequent and aggressive. When he turned three, Ari had a series of severe asthma attacks that required the liquid steroid my doctor had referred to as 'the atom bomb.'

The asthma specialist told me that he was a very sick boy who would need more and more medication just to maintain his airways. I simply couldn't face the prospect of standing over him for an endless stretch of nights, helplessly watching him struggle to breathe. That's when I decided to find another way of treating him.

When I first visited Dr. Linda Johnston, I had no idea what to expect. The duration and content of our meeting caught me totally off-guard. Not only had I never been asked for my observations about my son's mental and emotional state of being along with his physical symptoms, but I realised with a shock that I could no longer identify my son's 'healthy' state of being. I had known him as sick for so long, I thought the only standard of measuring his health was whether or not he struggled to breathe that day.

It was through Dr. Johnston's patient, thorough interviewing style that I understood for the first time that my son had become sick in more ways than just physically. In his case, the cure was almost as damaging as the disease; in one short year of asthma steroid treatment he had gone from outgoing and happy to moody, cautious and reserved. Dr. Johnston helped me realise that the personality changes that accompanied Ari's state of disease could be identified as part of his particular set of symptoms. Not only did this give me new hope for a better future for Ari's recovery, it also, equally importantly, gave me a new understanding of who my son truly was. He was a happy, outgoing boy when he was healthy. It was my obligation as a parent to restore him to his healthy state; his dreams, fears, food preferences, sleep patterns, and social behaviour were all clues for the doctor in evaluating his asthma case just as much or more as his actual wheezing and coughing.

Another new concept to me was that my son's physical symptoms were not meaningful in an absolute sense. I soon realised that after he had been given a remedy, Ari's symptoms would mimic his illness, but would be at a level that he could endure, and I didn't need to think of him as 'sick' during that time. Many times I called Dr. Johnston for help after a remedy, and she taught me the watchful waiting and observing that I find so useful to this day.

Once I was given to understand that there was an optimum state of wellness that my son could achieve, I then was able to grasp that I had the opportunity, as the doctor's home partner, to be able to identify when my son was slipping out of that state, so that I could bring him in to the doctor at the right time.

I also learned that my child didn't go from totally well to very sick in the blink of an eye; he had interim states, and those interim states followed a pattern each time his healthy energy started to slip. I developed a new paradigm for evaluating illness: I would observe the child's entire mental, emotional and physical state, and I would compare his altered state to the healthy standard that we had developed through homeopathic treatments. When Ari showed his familiar pattern of 'decline' behaviour, I could call Dr. Johnston to alert her that we'd probably be needing to see her in the next week or so, and through checking in on the phone with her over the next few days, we were able to pinpoint the best time for an office visit.

A most gratifying moment came several months into Ari's treatment, when, still at age three, he looked up at me out of the blue and said, 'I don't have asthma anymore, do I?' He felt 'well' for the first time in his memory. Now, at age ten, he is a very self-aware, self-confident boy who can articulate directly to the doctor how he is feeling, using the methods of observation that she taught us. Sometimes, when he's just not himself for a few days and seems to be at odds with his environment, I will ask him if it's time to go see Dr. Johnston. Even at ten, he knows when to say 'yes,' and when to say, 'let's watch for a few more days.'

Homeopathic medicine took me out of the passive role of blindly handing my child over to a doctor who only saw him briefly in his office once in a while, and instead deputised me into an active participant in assessing my child's symptoms. After all, since I was the one who lived with him twenty-four hours a day, it made sense that my home observations would be useful to enhance what the doctor could observe in a controlled office visit. The unexpected bonus is that it also made me a more connected parent. I am able to understand my children's temperaments, and offer them, beyond love and acceptance, actual understanding. Moreover, I have the peace of mind of knowing that they are maximising their potential in life by not wasting energy on trying to survive in a diseased state of being. By including me, the parent, in her diagnostic process, Dr. Johnston has enabled me to be a true partner in maintaining my children's health.'

Whose case is it?

The question often arises about how much of what a parent says should be taken into consideration. How much of what they say is their own state and how much is an objective assessment of the child? It is axiomatic that everything a person says, does and thinks comes from their inner state. It is impossible that it could be otherwise. Given that is the case, how can anyone ever describe anything or anyone except him or herself? It is simple; they cannot. Fortunately, however, this does not pose a problem in getting useful information about the child. It rests on our shoulders to perceive what is useful from a parent's report and what is not. Recall the cases in the previous chapters. In the case of Juglans cinerea, the mother's information was not as useful as was the mother's reports in the cases of Cimicifuga or Carboneum oxygenisatum. Making the determination of how much use parent's information will be is a case-by-case judgement call. I have found that the more informed the parent is about homeopathy and observing their child, the more reliable the information will be.

Peer pressure

Using homeopathy represents a different understanding of health, disease and symptoms, even a different view on life. As a result, sometimes a person choosing homeopathic treatment inadvertently becomes isolated from friends, relatives, teachers and peers. Not everyone is understanding or supportive of this choice. Even those who are interested in more natural ways of living, may draw the line when it comes to refusing conventional medical care for children.

It can be exceedingly difficult for the parent's relatives or friends who have no understanding of the process of homeopathy to watch a child go through a cold, runny nose, itching rash, sinus congestion or any other symptom. Their well-intended suggestions, advice, interventions and urging for 'proper' medical care for the child can be extremely problematic for the parent. It is hard enough in the best of circumstances to explain homeopathy, even to those eager to understand, let alone to opponents who see what they regard as a needlessly suffering child. The pressure on parents can be enormous. A homeopath should appreciate and be prepared to assist parents maintaining their choice even in the face of opposition from those important to them.

Much of the information in this book and in introductory books on homeopathy can be passed on to parents for the explicit purpose of helping them explain their choice should they need to. From my experience, it is difficult, if not impossible, for a parent to convince opponents what they are doing is right and valuable. This should not be a surprise. We as homeopaths are well aware of the near impenetrability of the conventional medical view and the staunch conviction of its adherents. I usually advise parents to refrain from engaging in debate and defensive arguments with people who are set out to convince them of how wrong they are to have homeopathic treatment. Instead, I encourage them to say something like, 'I really appreciate your interest and concern for me and my child. What would help me most right now is for you to acknowledge that I am an intelligent, informed adult, who loves my child and is wise enough to do what I think is best for him, even if you don't agree with my choices.' Sometimes the well-meaning person still insists on debating the issue, interfering with the parents' decisions or persisting in making the parents feel wrong or fearful about what they are doing. Another statement the parents can use is, 'I have asked you to respect me as an intelligent adult with my child's best interest at heart. If you cannot do that, I will no longer discuss this with you.'

There are circumstances in which schoolteachers have taken it upon themselves to make medical diagnoses and suggestions to parents, including insisting that the parents treat their child with psychotropic drugs such as those for depression, hyperactivity or attention deficit. A child being treated with homeopathy for hyperactivity, behaviour problems or other learning disabilities may cause their teacher extra work or stress because of the time it takes for the remedy to effect enough improvement to be demonstrable. Some teachers are very supportive and patient and others are not, some even demanding the parents immediately medicate their child as a condition of further schooling. Support of parents in these kinds of situations is essential. I have often had to remind teachers that they are not doctors and have no rights to intrude on parental decisions and medical choices.

Sometimes children are sent home from school with even minor symptoms and not allowed to return until their problems have been resolved. I have often written letters and made phone calls to school nurses or teachers to verify that the child is under my care and is not contagious or a danger to other children. I recall a particularly aware mother who brought her eight-year-old son with some nasal congestions and mild coughing of several days duration. The mother said, 'I know he doesn't really need to be seen because he is not that sick and will recover on his own. The problem is that the school is giving me a lot of hassle because I had not taken him to the doctor to get antibiotics.'

Hahnemann advises homeopaths to determine what is sick before deciding what to do about it. So it was with this case. The mother's diagnosis was quite correct; the problem was not with the child. He did not even need a dose of his remedy. It was the situation with the school staff that needed attention. Knowing that the boy was fine medically and it was perfectly safe for all concerned for him to return to school, I needed to reassure the staff in a way meaningful to them. I wrote 'penicillin' on a piece of paper and pinned it to the boy's shirt and sent him back. Neither the mother nor I heard another word.

In the last chapter, immunisations were discussed at length to provide useful information to pass along to parents grappling with this issue. Even for parents who have firmly decided not to immunise, there can be a question about a school's entrance requirement for immunisations. I can only speak with certainty of the situation in the United States, but other countries' policies may be similar. Many parents are purposely led to believe that it is an inescapable legal requirement for a child to have all mandatory immunisations before he can attend school and they have no choice in the matter. School nurses and other officials promote the idea that this is the law. It is not the law. Though an extremely well kept secret, the law does not override parental rights by forcing them to immunise their child against their will. The laws in all 50 states in the USA allow for a medical exemption to being immunised. The letter I write for parents to meet the requirement and allow their child to enter school is, '(Child's name) has been under my medical care for (months or years). It is against my medical advice for him to have immunisations.' It has not been necessary to add anything further. This letter has always been accepted and no child under my care has ever been refused school admission because of lack of immunisations.

Dealing with allopathic medical doctors

In the course of treating children sometimes it is necessary to interact with conventional medical doctors. An orthopaedic doctor needs to set a broken arm, a surgeon needs to remove an inflamed appendix or other occasions arise in which an allopath's services are needed. More commonly, when the child first comes to the homeopath, he already has doctors he has visited for medical care. Depending on the medical condition being treated, these could include rheumatologists, nephrologists, neurologists or any other specialty. Some of these doctors are accepting of the idea of homeopathic treatment and others can be downright hostile, placing the parent in an untenable and stressful situation. There are two areas to examine; one is the homeopath interacting with doctors and the other is the parents' relationship with their child's other doctors.

One way or another, it does happen that homeopaths will interface with medical doctors. If the homeopath is also a medical doctor, it can be easier than if the homeopath is a non-medical doctor such as a chiropractor, naturopath or unlicensed lay practitioner. Even as a medical doctor, I have occasionally had unpleasant situations when having to interact with the child's other doctor. Fortunately these have been rare. The most distressing situation was one in which a particularly ill eight-year-old child was placed in my care. After six months of careful homeopathic treatment, her serious chronic disease had shown remarkable improvement. Not only had her symptoms resolved but she also no longer needed prescription medications and she grew 5 cm (2 in) and a shoe size! The mother was so delighted with the successful outcome with homeopathy that she insisted that she wanted to share news of this miraculous improvement with the child's former specialist. As soon as the mother brought the child into the specialist's office, he was delighted and amazed at her change. He exclaimed to the mother, 'You see, I told you I would get her better! All you had to do is follow my treatment program. She looks wonderful.' Perplexed, the child looked up at the mother. After one of those pregnant pauses, the girl said, 'But doctor, I have not been taking your medicines.'

Now the doctor was perplexed. He asked the mother to explain, which she did. She had stopped his treatment and for six months had only homeopathic treatment. If a sunny day can turn to a gale storm in the flash of an eye, so did this doctor. He was furious and began berating the mother about the dangerous course she had taken with her daughter's precarious medical condition. After his lengthy tirade, his parting shot was to inform the mother he was going to start legal proceedings to have the child removed from her because she was unfit to make medical decisions for the child. Imagine how upset she was! She honestly thought the doctor would be happy the child was improved, rather than threatened and threatening because she dared to question his authority. Though the doctor's threats turned out to be empty ones, the mother was frightened for months to come.

Though this was the most extreme case I have encountered, there have been a few occasions in which the other doctor refuses to continue to participate in the child's care as long as he is under homeopathic treatment. Fortunately, most of the time, when another doctor is involved, a productive collaboration is worked out. There is no hard and fast rule about how to interact with other doctors; each is different and each situation is different. Whatever the case, a homeopath will be confronted with the need to deal with many kinds of different doctors, who have a wide range of attitudes towards homeopathy and homeopathic treatment.

The parent also may have occasion to interact with other doctors, psychologists or therapists. Some parents prefer to discuss openly with all physicians involved in the child's care and others prefer to keep information about the homeopathic treatment separate and undisclosed. This depends entirely on the character of the parent and the other medical personnel they come in contact with. I follow the parents' lead and participate with other practitioners and doctors to whatever degree they desire.

Remedy information

Many parents have told me that one of the most useful things I do is to assist them in understanding their child better by explaining the themes and character of their child's remedy. This is also beneficial because I can inform the parents about the kinds of stresses and situations to which their child is most sensitive. For example, the parent of a Lycopodium child can be alert for signs of illness when their child will be performing or starting a new school, situations that are particularly stressful for Lycopodium. The parents of a Calcarea carbonica child can be attentive to keeping the household environment as stable as possible, and watch for signs of illness when there are major disruptions to household routine. Of course, in a healthy state, each child should be able to cope with any of these events. However, the nature of the remedy that works for the child will determine which situations may deplete their inner resources more quickly. This information is very useful for the parents to have.

An interesting example is the remedy Magnesium carbonicum. The theme and character of this remedy is to feel like a helpless infant, dependent on others for care, food, warmth and shelter coupled with the urge and desire to exert his own choices. But he fears that if he does express his own desire, those he is dependent on will forsake and abandon him and he will be left alone, like an orphan without loving attention, enough nourishment or proper shelter. That prospect is so frightening that he suppresses himself, and becomes what others want him to be. He cannot be himself; he cannot have his own identity.

If the fear of losing those on whom he is dependent were the only issue, the person would simply remain contently dependent catering to their wishes in exchange for a secure relationship, which provides for his needs. On the other hand, if expressing one's desires and choices were the only issue, the person would do just that, irrespective of the consequences. The conflict and tension for Magnesium carbonicum arises because both drives are operating at the same time. The urge to have an identity, make choices, have one's own personality is opposed by his helpless dependency on others for care and nourishment. This ever-present urge for self-expression combined with the fear of being abandoned because one did so creates the problem, the catch-22. His constant fear of being abandoned is because the urge for self-expression is indwelling and constant. He is frightened of the inevitable abandonment should that desire burst out, escaping its suppression.

Think of a child needing Magnesium carbonicum. The child clings to her parents, is fearful and timid. She always asks, 'Mommy, do you love me?' or declares, 'Mommy, you don't love me!' She has dreams of being kidnapped, of baby animals with their mothers and being fed by them. Explaining the inner world of this child to her parents, the homeopath must help the parents understand that the child's inner world is not necessarily related to the reality of the situation. This is a critical point, otherwise these loving, caring parents would find it impossible to understand why their daughter lives in a world in which she feels abandoned like an orphan, whose parents have forsaken her so she is without love and enough food or proper shelter. Once the parents understand that this is the inner world from which the child experiences life, their child's behaviour and reactions start to make sense. It is understandable why an orphan child would constantly ask if her mother loved her. The dream of a mother animal feeding its young exemplifies the opposite of her feelings – she has no mother and is not fed. Stepping into their child's inner world, the parents can understand and support the child effectively as well as be alert to signs when another dose of the remedy is needed.

There is no blame

Parents often ask me where these ideas of their child come from? In the situation above, parents would ask where did the idea of being forsaken or alone come from? They want to know why their child feels the way they do. The parents want to know if it was something they did or neglected to do that created these inexplicable feelings and thoughts that occupy their child's inner world. Additionally, when there is a connection between the mother's state in pregnancy and the child's symptoms, the mother wants to know what she did to make her child sick.

Why man becomes sick is an age-old question, to which there is no definitive answer. It is not known why anyone has a particular foreign energy interfering with his healthy, normal energy state. Why a specific child is in a particular energy state is also unanswerable. Though it is not known why an adult or child becomes sick, it is certainly not the parents' fault. It is very important to emphasise this point to parents, especially when the mother worries that traumatic or stressful events during her pregnancy may have harmed her child. As parents become more aware of the homeopathic perspective, they can become guilt ridden for having previously given their child antibiotics, steroids or other medications and immunisations. The homeopath must reassure the parents that they are not to blame for anything. No doubt, the parents have always been caring and concerned, wanting the very best for their child, and should be commended for now seeking out a better way to keep their child healthy. Nothing can change the past, but the very fact they are in the homeopath's office is a testament to their continual search to help their child in every possible way.

What not why

Most parents think they know and understand their children very well. For the most part, they do. However, it is often the case that parents are surprised by the things their child has said during the homeopathic case-taking. The loving parents of the above Magnesium carbonicum child had no idea their child felt like an orphan. Equally surprising is how the homeopath can elicit such hidden inner thoughts and feelings when the parents have not.

Homeopaths and parents listen to the child from very different points of view. Their goals are different from each other. A homeopath hears these inner thoughts because he knows they are there, and focuses his inquiry in that direction. He knows there is another energy expressing itself, usually hidden, suppressed and compensated. In the case of children, it can be as simple as the fact that no one has taken the time to listen to them intently, without judging or correcting them.

Parents want to understand their child and to be able to hear the same things that the homeopath does. My suggestion to parents is to listen closely and intently, focusing on the question, 'what', not 'why'. As was previously discussed, understanding a person can be achieved by hearing them describe what their personal experience is. It is not helpful for them to explain why it is. The same is true for parents talking with their child. To enter the child's world, the password is 'what', then staying quiet to hear the amazing story of his inner world unfold.

Conclusion

Working with parents, educating them, deputising them, involving them adds a wonderful and enjoyable dimension to the usual treatment of children. I encourage each homeopath to take the time to involve parents as much as possible. If you ever doubt the usefulness of this approach, reread Rachel Lipman Mostow's description of her experience. An involved parent and a healthy child make a winning team.

The purpose of this book has been to open up a whole new world of possibilities, excitement, success and fulfilment in the treatment of children by exploring the new methods and ideas in homeopathy. There is no reward quite like the feeling of successfully treating a child, knowing that his improved health will make a positive difference in the trajectory of his life for its entire duration. Watching these children grow, develop their individuality and face life's challenges with strength, curiosity and joy is the best part of being a homeopath.

This book is just the opening chapter in the use of new methods for the treatment of children. To apply the methods and ideas that have been introduced, it will be helpful to study them in more detail and practice them in the clinic. Certainly more knowledge of materia medica and philosophy will be useful. The most important part, however, is the most enjoyable – talking to children. By creating a safe, calm rapport, with keen interest, patience and an accepting approach, the homeopath can enjoy the wondrous, amazing and surprising journey through the child's world.

INDEX

accidents 181–182

Aconitum 9

acute disease 14

Adamas 123–125
  see diamond

Adler, Mortimer 36

adoption 178–179

aetiology and vulnability 177–178

allergies 86–107, 129, 130, 134, 183, 192

allergic rhinitis 129, 135

allopathic doctors, dealing with
  197–198

Anand, Sunnil 19, 81, 115–123, 138–150,
  155–165

Androctonus 166, 170

Antimonium crudum 15

aphorism 23, 24

Aristotle 68

approach to treating children 1–5
  traditional approach 7–16
  new approach 19–32
  see source-based prescribing

Arnica 9, 13, 128

Artichoke
  see Cynara scolymus

Asteraceae 128

asthma 21, 86–107, 192–194

Baryta carbonica 156

being stuck 25–26, 147

Bellis perennis 128

birth 8, 33, 34, 42–47, 59–65, 70

black cohosh
  see Cimicifuga racemosa

blastospheres 8

Borax 146

Borland, Douglas M 7

breath, breathing 26, 55, 59, 62, 88, 97,
  100, 141, 143, 146, 153, 161

Bryce, James 11

caesarean section 151, 166, 168, 170, 172

Calcaria carbonica 15, 97, 99, 198

Calendula 128

Carbo oxygenisatum 149

Carbo veg 124

Carbon 122, 124, 147

Carbon dioxide 124

carbon monoxide
  see Carbon oxygenisatum

Carbon oxygenisatum 147–148, 194

carboneum salts 124

carbonicum salts 124

carbonous oxide
  see Carbo oxygenisatum

Carduus 128

cases
  a patient's perspective 192–194
  asthma 86–107
  child in utero reveals the source
    166–174
  dream reveals the source 150–156
  dreaming of the source 125–129
  keynote prescribing 14–15
  lack of imagination 54–55
  living with the source 129–135
  mother reveals the source 157–166
  naming the source 115–125
  pregnancy reveals the source 138–150
  source words 110
  telephone consultation 13
  treating asthma 21

case taking 11, 23, 24, 77-83
  confidence 79-80
  in asthma 21
  more methods 107-108
  parent input 194
  source words 101, 110, 145, 164-166
Causa occasionalis 176
Cenchris 155
Center for Disease Control 183
Chhabra, Divya 19, 20, 27, 28
chickenpox 15
chief complaint 81-82
Childhood 33-34, 74
  see development, childhood
children's types 3, 7-8, 9, 83
child's world, entering 51-52, 77-78
Chocolate 21
chronic disease 14
Cichoriodeae 128
Cimicifuga racemosa 163-164, 194
Cina 139
coeliac disease 81, 138, 139
colds and flu 14, 30, 87, 118, 146, 156,
  162
commonality 1, 9
compensated patient 28-29
cough 12, 13, 88-96, 103, 104, 162
Cynaria scolymus 126-127, 128, 129

Descartes, René 55, 72
development, brain 44-48
  brain function 46-48
  brain growth 44-46
  brain structure 46-47
    brain stem 46
    cerebellum 47
    cerebrum 47
    limbic area 47
    midbrain 46-47
    old brain
      see brain stem
    reticular formations 47
development, childhood 34-38, 65-74
  newborn 8, 62-65
  first year of life 65-66
  aged one to four 66-69

aged four 69-71
aged four to seven 71-72
aged seven to eleven 72-73
aged 11-14 73-74
normal development 25-26, 27, 31, 35
development, emotional 34, 36, 44, 54,
  66, 67, 68, 74
development, mental
  childhood imagination 47, 51, 55-58,
    71, 72, 73
  childhood learning 33, 36, 38, 39, 41,
    44, 45, 51, 53-58, 64, 68, 69, 71
  childhood logic 51, 52, 53-58, 60, 70,
    71, 72, 73, 74
  childhood play 34, 40, 50, 52-58,
    70-73
  enviromental stimulation 35, 36, 40,
    45, 54, 56, 60, 62, 63, 65-67
  innate timetable 57-58
  sensory understanding 49, 52, 55, 60,
    73
  time perception 58-62
  verbal ability 1, 178
development, neurological 39, 44, 45, 46,
  48, 49, 56, 58, 60, 62, 64, 66, 70
development, normal 25-26, 27, 31,
  34-35, 37, 43, 46, 50, 55, 56, 63,
  74
development, physical 33, 34, 36, 37, 38,
  39-43, 52
  standing 39, 58
  teething 41-43, 67, 139
  walking 38, 40-41, 44, 58, 67
development, physiological 59, 63, 64
development, social 180
developmental cycle 35, 37
diamond 119, 120, 121-123, 124
  Koh-i-Noor 117, 121, 122
  see Adamas
Diphtherinum 183
discrimination 24
disease 2, 7, 10, 14, 23, 28, 29, 30, 80, 81,
  115, 125, 126, 138, 139, 177, 182, 183,
  185, 186, 187, 188, 191, 193, 194,
  195, 197
doodle 138, 159, 164-165

dreams 97, 104, 120, 126–127, 131–132,
    144, 150–156, 168, 170, 171

ear infection 30, 157, 162
eco-system 4
eczema 151, 155
Eising, Nuala 20
embryogenesis 8
energy 22–30, 34–37, 43, 70, 82–84, 92,
    134, 136, 137, 140, 147, 148, 157, 158,
    160–163, 165, 167, 168, 175, 176,
    183, 193, 194, 200
  energy field 22, 24, 84, 175
  energy source 22–27, 78–79, 83–85,
    111, 132, 175, 176
  energy state see energy field
  energy, vital 29–30, 34–35
Eupatorium 128
Euphorbiaceae 26
expressing individuality 113–114

family dynamics 179–180
family themes
  see group themes
fantasy 53
Fluoric acid 173–174
Franklin, Benjamin 38

gestures 142, 143, 157, 158, 159, 160, 163,
    165, 166
getting started 5
group themes 28
Ginott, Dr Haim 177
Graphites 124
Grimes, Melanie 20
growth 33, 38, 41, 42, 43–44, 48, 52, 54,
    56, 64, 69, 72, 73, 74
  brain growth 44–46, 52, 53, 62

Hahnemann, Samuel 2, 16, 20, 23, 24, 35,
    77, 80, 114, 176, 196
  see aphorisms & Organon
Hamamelidae 101, 102
head
  aches 116, 117, 125, 126, 127, 128, 129,
    134, 135

spinning sensation 90, 91, 93, 95, 96
health 2–4, 14, 19, 22, 23, 24–27, 29, 31,
    34–37, 42, 43, 50, 54, 64, 68, 69, 77,
    88, 130, 138, 143, 147, 176–178, 180,
    187, 193–195, 198, 200, 201
Heller, Joseph 27
Hering, Constantine 20,155
homeopathy in America 7

immunisations 88, 161, 182–188, 196
importance of difference 49–51
individuality 8, 9
inner conflict 26–28
insects, fear of 130–131
inter-uterine life 59, 62
irritable bowel syndrome (IBS) 162

Jenner, Edward 183
Joshi, Bhawisha 124
Juglans cinerea 102, 106
Julian, Dr 20
Jung, Carl Gustav 4

KeBoyer, Frederick 65
Keller, Helen 112
keynote prescribing 3, 10–11, 14–15, 16
Klein, Louis 20
König, Peter 20
Kreosote 124

Lac caninum 109
Lac felinum 109
Lachesis 155
Latrodectus mactans 134–135
Linnaeus, Carolus 112
Lithium 26
Lycopodium 198

Magnesium carbonicum 198
Magnesium phosphoricum 125
Malvaceae 26
marriage 8
Maslow, Abraham 37
materia medica 12, 16, 20, 21, 103, 110,
    124, 128, 200
Mezger, Dr 20

miasm 97, 102, 161, 163, 164
Mumbai 78-79
moving 55-56, 81, 138, 140, 145, 146,
        147, 148, 149
Müller, Karl Joseph 20

Natrum muriaticum 27
'never well since' 177
Nitrogen 146
Norland, Misha 20
nutmeg 109

observation 11, 12
Onopordon 128
Opium 171, 172
Organon of Medicine 16, 19, 35
        see Hahnemann, Samuel & aphorisms
orthodontic braces 181
Oxygen 147

parents and parenting 4-5, 12, 14, 15, 23,
        35, 39, 40, 44, 50, 51, 53, 57, 58, 63,
        68, 69, 72, 85, 86, 87, 88, 99, 101, 112,
        121, 176, 178, 180, 182, 185,
        191-200
    deputised parent 5, 191-192, 194
    explaining remedy to parent 198-199
    immunisation and parents 182-188
    see allopathic doctors - dealing with
patient undivided attention 85-86
pathognomonic 10
peculiar symptoms 23, 24, 83
peer pressure 195-197
periodic table 37
Pertussinum 183
Petroleum 124
Phelps, William Lyon 51
Potter, Harry 51-52
pregnancy 87, 118, 137, 138, 141, 144,
        145, 150-152, 154, 161, 168,
        170-172
provings 20, 21, 84, 122, 124

Raeside, Dr 20
repertory 114
    Kent 13

repertorisation 9-10
Reynolds, Sir Joshua 11
Riley, David 20
Rowe, Todd 20
rubrics 10, 13, 15, 26, 41, 42, 56, 61, 102,
        114, 148, 171, 173

Saccharum 124
Sankaran, Rajan 19, 20, 28, 97, 101, 102,
        124, 163
Santayana, George 72
Santos, Uta 20
Schadde, Anne 20
Schuster, Bernd 20
sensation-based prescribing
    see source-based prescribing
Seuss, Dr 4
Shah, Jayesh 19, 20, 28, 124
Sherr, Jeremy 20, 21
Shore, Jonathan 20
Shukla, Chetna 20
siblings 63, 128, 175, 179, 180
simillimum 21, 23, 183
snake remedies 154-155
Souk-Aloun, Dr 20
source of remedies 22
source-based prescribing 3, 19-20, 21,
        22-23, 26, 30, 31, 77, 86, 109
    cases 86-107, 115-135, 138-174
    methods and techniques 77-109
    power of names 111-112
    remedy as symbol 114-115
    source words 110-111, 127, 132
    words as symbol 112
spring water 143, 147
Stramonium 29
Strange symptoms
    see peculiar symptoms
stress 63-64
sulphur 109
Swan, Dr 147

Taraxicum 128
Theory of Relativity 59
time vision, depth of 58-61
totality of symptoms 15, 23

traditional methods 2, 3, 7, 23
    see approach to treating children
treatment goal 2, 19
Tunerculinum 183

understanding the child neurologically
    48–49
unusual symptons
    see peculiar symptoms
upper respiratory tract infection 157

Vaccine Injury Compensation Program
    186
vaccines 183
van der Zee, Harry 124
Variolinum 183

White, T.H. 84
Wilson's disease 115, 125
Wordsworth, William 4